Complete Dentures
From Planning to Problem Solving

Quintessentials of Dental Practice – 12
Prosthodontics - 2

Complete Dentures

From Planning to Problem Solving

By
P Finbarr Allen
Seán McCarthy

Editor-in-Chief: Nairn H F Wilson
Editor Prosthodontics: P Finbarr Allen

Quintessence Publishing Co. Ltd.

London, Berlin, Chicago, Copenhagen, Paris, Milan, Barcelona,
Istanbul, São Paulo, Tokyo, New Dehli, Moscow, Prague, Warsaw

British Library Cataloguing in Publication Data

Allen, P. Finbarr
    Complete dentures : from planning to problem solving. –
    (The quintessentials of dental practice ; 12. Prosthodontics ; 2)
    1. Complete dentures
    I. Title II. McCarthy, Seán
    617.6'92

ISBN 1850970645

ISBN 1-85097-064-5

Dedicated to our families and our patients.

Foreword

The clinical and technical challenges in successful complete denture prostho-dontics are many and varied. Assisting patients in the transition to complete dentures and giving edentulous patients dental comfort and confidence is a very demanding but rewarding aspect of clinical practice. However, many patients seeking immediate and replacement complete dentures present with a long history of dissatisfaction and discomfort with dentures, a feeling of being "dentally disabled", and a plethora of emotions ranging from embar-rassment to frank distress over their edentulousness and reliance on remov-able dental prostheses.

The tense, tight-lipped, stern-looking lady gripping the bag of failed com-plete dentures and reading the practice pamphlet on complaints as she waits impatiently for her first appointment with you is a daunting sight. But even these cases can be managed successfully by a careful, systematic approach to complete denture provision. *Complete Dentures: From Planning to Problem Solv-ing* - the eleventh volume in the Quintessentials of Dental Practice Series - describes and illustrates this approach in the now familiar, easy-to-read style of the Quintessentials Series. Starting with "the countdown to edentulous-ness" and running all the way through to "the shifting treatment paradigm: replacement dentures or implant-retained prostheses", this attractive book is packed with practical advice for the general dental practitioner. Notwith-standing the clinical procedures and skills necessary to meet the needs and expectations of patients requiring complete dentures, special emphasis is placed on communication and team working with the dental technician.

If your dentures could be in the stern-looking lady's bag of failed dentures, then this book will be a most valuable addition to your dental library.

Nairn Wilson
Editor-in-Chief

Editor's Foreword

Rehabilitation of edentulous patients is one of the mainstays of general dental practice. In this second volume for the Prosthodontics section of the Quintessentials for Dental Practitioners series, the authors address the management of edentulous patients. Both authors have extensive clinical experience at primary and secondary care level and use their experience to inform the approach to problem solving for edentulous patients.

Each chapter is prefaced by aims and anticipated outcomes, and key clinical points and conclusions are presented at the end of the chapters. High-quality clinical illustrations are used to demonstrate clinical techniques and to help guide practitioners, members of the dental team and undergraduate students.

As the population ages, there is a significant problem with older adults losing their natural teeth at a time when they are unlikely to adapt to wearing complete dentures. The authors deal with this issue first, and describe techniques which will help the practitioner manage the transition to edentulousness successfully. Planning and problem solving for complete replacement dentures is discussed with the emphasis on treatment planning rather than a recipe book approach to denture construction. Finally, the role of implant-retained prostheses is discussed. This book is recommended for all students and general practitioners and will help foster a thoughtful approach to the management of edentulous patients.

P Finbarr Allen

Preface

Provision of complete dentures was a significant component of the undergraduate dental curriculum and of general dental practice. Improvements in dental health have reduced this requirement, but large numbers of edentate patients are still present in the population. Furthermore, the proportion of elderly adults is rapidly increasing as life expectancy increases. Many of these adults will not retain sufficient teeth, and will require complete dentures at some point in their lives. The first chapter of this book deals with the management of the transition to the edentulous state. This is a critical period for the older adult with a failing natural dentition, and many of the problems associated with failure to adapt to complete dentures arise at this stage. If the transition is managed carefully using good prosthetic technique, and the patient and dentist have a shared vision of the treatment goal, then subsequent problems can be avoided. The bulk of the text deals with the planning, construction and review of complete dentures. Emphasis is placed on customising the treatment plan to the individual patient's requirements and each chapter should be considered as a part of a continuum rather than completely free-standing. Finally, the influence of osseointegrated prostheses in the management of edentulism is discussed in the last chapter. This form of treatment has been a major advance in prosthetic dentistry, but should it be seen as the "gold standard" of treatment for the edentulous state?

Having Read This Book

It is hoped that having read this book the reader will be able to:
- Recognise the desirability of avoiding total tooth loss in old age.
- Understand that, when total tooth loss is inevitable, the transition to edentulousness should be made in a co-ordinated manner.
- Plan treatment for an edentulous patient, bearing in mind the huge variety in presentation of these patients.
- Recognise the relationship between retention, stability and support, and the impact of this relationship on complete denture technique.
- Follow a systematic approach to problem solving in patients with difficulties wearing complete dentures.
- Understand the role of implant-retained overdentures in the management of edentulous patients.

Contents

Chapter 1
Countdown to Edentulousness: Managing the Transition Successfully

Aim

The aim of this chapter is to describe how the transition to the edentulous state can be managed successfully.

Outcome

At the end of this chapter, the clinician should be aware that the loss of all natural teeth in old age is undesirable. It should be recognised that maintenance of a healthy, functioning natural dentition for life is the ideal goal for older adults. The prognosis for the natural dentition should be monitored and if total tooth loss becomes inevitable, then a gradual transition to the edentulous state should be planned. The practitioner should be aware of the various strategies possible for achieving this, beginning with the use of transitional removable partial dentures.

Introduction

A substantial body of evidence exists in the scientific literature, which documents the sequelae of total tooth loss. Although the number of adults losing their natural teeth is diminishing, there are still large numbers of edentulous adults in the population. This situation is likely to continue for many years to come, as the generation of adults rendered edentulous early in life ages. If a dentist can successfully rehabilitate edentulous patients, especially those with denture-wearing difficulties, then this will have a positive influence on the perception of their practice. Increasingly, the impact of poor quality diet on general health has been emphasised, and loss of teeth has an influence on this. Dentists have an important role to play in providing good quality complete dentures and in encouraging their edentulous patients to improve the quality of their diet. In addition to successfully managing the problems of the edentulous patient, a further requirement is to manage the transition to edentulousness. As the problems of older adults with an ageing dentition have become more challenging, it is vital that the clinician anticipates problems and plans dental care accordingly.

Adult Dental Health Trends

Population surveys of adult dental health indicate that older adults are retaining their teeth longer, and that the prevalence of edentulousness is decreasing rapidly. However, there are many threats to tooth retention, and there has been a shift towards total tooth loss occurring later in life. Clinical experience suggests that successful adaptation to edentulousness is less predictable in old age, as the ability to develop the complex skills required to control complete replacement dentures diminishes with age.

As well as the decrease in edentulousness, population surveys also indicate that there is a high level of dental disease in older adults, particularly loss of periodontal attachment and root surface caries. A further problem is the cumulative sequelae of a lifetime of the treatment of disease and of large restorations. For the most part, the increased retention of teeth in older adults is not as a result of lower levels of disease but of higher levels of treatment. For many, the goal of retaining teeth in old age may be beyond reach, and total tooth loss may be inevitable. Consequently, major challenges for dentists include:

- Predicting the likelihood of their patients retaining teeth into old age and recognising the threats to this ideal goal.
- Planning care based on retaining sufficient numbers of teeth for satisfactory oral function.
- Managing the transition to the edentulous state when retention of teeth seems unlikely.

Edentulous Maxilla Opposing Partially Dentate Mandible

At the present time, large numbers of adults have edentate maxillary arches opposed by partially dentate mandibular arches. Further clinical presentations include partially dentate adults with unrestored tooth spaces. These patients may lose the remainder of the natural dentition late in life, and they present a significant management challenge to dentists. They may have a removable partial denture to replace posterior teeth, but in many cases they do not have a mandibular prosthesis. A common problem when such a combination presents is that of "flabby" tissue in the anterior maxilla. This may make the maxillary complete denture unstable, because the flabby tissue displaces during function. The problem of the displaceable ("flabby") anterior ridge is discussed in more detail in Chapter 3. A further difficulty may be that there are insufficient occlusal contacts to maintain a stable maxillary denture. When molar and premolar teeth are missing, occlusal forces are directed through the anterior aspect of the maxillary denture, resulting in a tipping force which displaces the denture posteriorly. The clinical challenge is to decide how many occlusal contacts are required to overcome this situation, and this varies from patient to patient. In addition to making a complete maxillary denture, the following treatment options for the mandible should be considered:

- Accepting that the number of natural mandibular teeth present is sufficient, and aim to balance the occlusion using a semi-adjustable articulator to construct the maxillary denture.
- Restoring missing teeth with a removable partial denture (RPD).
- Extending the shortened dental arch using cantilevered bridgework. Conventional retainers can be used if the last standing teeth are heavily restored or resin-bonded bridges can be used if the teeth are unrestored.
- Extending shortened dental arches with implant-retained crowns or bridges.

There are a number of factors to consider when deciding which of these options is appropriate for the patient. If the maxillary complete denture is stable, then it is likely that the patient has sufficient occlusal contacts, and preserving the mandibular dentition without a prosthesis is indicated. The clinician must also bear in mind that there should be a good long-term prognosis for the remaining mandibular teeth when choosing this option. If further teeth are lost at a later date, this may compromise the patient's ability to wear a removable prosthesis. Consequently, this treatment option is contraindicated if the remaining natural teeth are mobile, have significant (>5 mm) pocketing or show signs of advanced tooth wear (Fig 1-1).

Removable partial dentures are widely used, but bilateral, unbounded (free-end) dentures are frequently discarded. In many cases, they are poorly con-

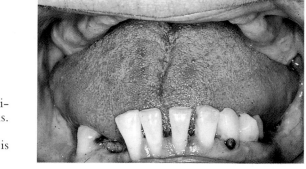

Fig 1-1 Mandibular dentition with a poor prognosis. Application of the shortened dental arch concept is contraindicated.

structed, and this is a significant influence on poor compliance by the patient. Factors which may improve tolerance of bilateral free-end saddle dentures include: (a) using the RPI system of clasp design to reduce torque forces on abutment teeth; (b) using the altered cast impression technique to reduce sinking of the saddle areas of the denture into the underlying tissues; (c) reducing the size of the occlusal table to reduce the load transmitted to the underlying ridges. In some cases, despite the use of good clinical technique, the patient feels uncomfortable and discards the denture.

If the mandibular dental arch extends to the first premolar teeth, and if the patient has had difficulty with a removable partial denture, the arch can be extended by one premolar unit on each side using *bridgework*. This will increase the number of posterior occlusal contacts thereby increasing the stability of the maxillary denture. There should be a good prognosis for the remaining teeth when considering this treatment option. Full coverage retainers are indicated if large restorations are present in the abutment teeth, and the size and design of the pontic should be the subject of careful consideration. If the abutment tooth is unrestored, then a resin–bonded bridge can be used. Clinical research indicates that success with this option increases if preparation features such as proximal grooves and rest seats are present. When bonding these bridges to teeth, rubber dam isolation is recommended.

Implant-retained restorations are expensive and involve surgical procedures. Care must also be taken to avoid damage to anatomical structure during surgery. It is debatable whether these restorations offer significant advantages when compared with bridgework in this clinical scenario. Patient preference may tip the balance in favour of implants but, as with bridgework, there should be a favourable prognosis for the remainder of the natural dentition when considering this treatment option.

Limiting treatment goals to provide a shortened dental arch (SDA), or extending an SDA with cantilevered bridgework will provide a suboptimal, but probably acceptable, level of function. However, there should be a favourable long-term prognosis for the remaining natural dentition, as loss of these teeth later in life may compromise a successful transition to wearing a complete denture. The various options for managing the edentulous maxilla opposed by a natural dentition are summarised in Table 1-1.

Table 1-1 Treatment options and their indications for managing a mandibular shortened dental arch opposed by a maxillary complete denture.

RPD	SDA	Bridgework	Implants
canines, incisors present	stable upper denture	premolars, canines, incisors present	premolars, canines, incisors present
?prognosis for remaining teeth	good prognosis for remaining teeth	good prognosis for remaining teeth	good prognosis for remaining teeth
		intolerance of RPD	intolerance of RPD
			patient preference

RPD, removable partial denture; SDA, shortened dental arch.

The Dentition With a Poor Prognosis – Stages in the Transition To Edentulousness

If at all possible, the loss of teeth in old age should be avoided. Ideally, if the patient is a regular attender, the dentist can then make an assessment of the prognosis of the remaining dentition. If the patient has active periodontal disease which has failed to respond to treatment, then total tooth loss is likely. Further threats are dental caries and pathological tooth wear. Patients may also dislike the appearance of their natural dentition and may request a dental clearance. This may not be an unreasonable request, but the patient should be made aware of the possible consequences of this action. The decision to render a patient edentulous should not be taken lightly in view of the potential adverse consequences of edentulousness, including the following:

- resorption of the residual alveolar ridge
- reduced chewing efficiency
- limitation of food selection, especially nutritious foods such as fruits and vegetables
- speech impairment
- change in appearance
- psychosocial impact.

When it is recognised that the prognosis for the remaining dentition is poor, this should be communicated to the patient and possible treatment strategies discussed carefully. A key factor in ensuring a successful treatment outcome is that the patient understands and accepts the goals of treatment. Patient input and a feeling of "ownership" of the process is, therefore, essential.

There are three possible scenarios for the dentist:
1. The patient is a regular attender and a gradual transition to edentulousness can be made.
2. The patient is not a regular attender, but accepts that the prognosis for their remaining teeth is poor and is prepared to make a gradual transition to edentulousness.
3. The patient is not a regular attender, and upon initial presentation, tooth loss is inevitable and imminent.

Caries, periodontal disease and pathological tooth wear are the disease processes likely to lead to total tooth loss.

Terminal dentition – caries and periodontal disease

If the remaining dentition is severely affected by periodontal disease or dental caries, then gradual tooth loss leading to complete replacement dentures is indicated. In scenario 1, the transition to edentulousness can be managed in a controlled fashion. If the patient has no previous denture-wearing experience, then transitional removable partial dentures should be prescribed. The purpose of a transitional denture is:
1. to allow the patient the opportunity to accommodate to wearing dentures
2. to minimise the encroachment of the tongue into the space vacated by extraction of the posterior teeth and
3. to facilitate gradual addition of teeth as the patient loses more natural teeth.

It is absolutely critical that transitional dentures are constructed carefully, as rejection of these dentures may compromise eventual acceptance of complete replacement dentures. Consequently, they should be designed to be as retentive and stable as possible (Fig 1-2). The patient in Fig 1-3 is an example of a gradual transition to the edentulous state. She had caries and periodontal disease which did not respond to treatment, and it was decided to gradually render her edentulous. She was provided with acrylic, tissue-borne transitional partial dentures with wrought stainless steel clasps in the first instance. After some months of successful wearing of these dentures, impressions were made of the dentures in situ using irreversible hydrocolloid. In the laboratory, the casts were poured and the dentures located to the remaining natural teeth on the casts. The natural teeth were removed from the casts and denture teeth added to convert the partial denture to a complete denture. In the clinic, the remaining natural teeth were extracted and the complete dentures inserted.

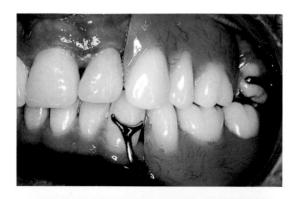

Fig 1-2 Transitional partial dentures with clasps.

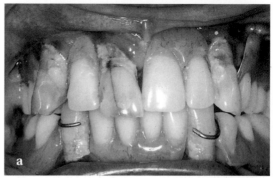

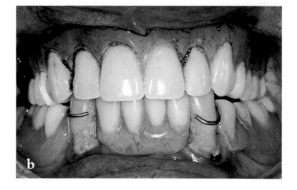

Fig 1-3 (a) Transitional partial denture to which teeth have been added gradually; (b) after extraction of the remaining teeth, it has been converted to a complete denture.

Terminal dentition – pathological tooth wear

A further possibility is to use the roots of the natural teeth to support a partial overdenture, and this can be used in tooth wear cases or where teeth are too broken down to retain crowns. In this situation, the teeth identified as

suitable for overdenture abutments should be prepared. Criteria for overdenture abutments are:
- at least two roots should be retained
- the roots should be symmetrically distributed
- it should be possible to create a coronal dome with or without restorations
- at least 50% bone support remains
- endodontic procedures should be possible.

A number of benefits can accrue from maintaining the roots, such as preservation of alveolar bone, aiding the stability and retention of dentures, psychological well-being and maintenance of proprioception.

Transitional partial dentures can be made initially to replace missing teeth and overlay worn tooth surfaces to improve appearance and restore occlusal face height (Fig 1-4). After a suitable period of wearing transitional partial dentures, such prostheses can be converted to complete overdentures. This can be achieved by:
1. Recording an impression of the partial denture in situ and asking the dental technician to prepare the remaining natural teeth on the model cast from this impression. When the denture is returned, the clinician trims the teeth to a dome shape, and modifies the fitting surface of the denture with self-cure acrylic resin to fit the prepared teeth.
2. Recording an impression of the denture in situ and then cutting the natural teeth to a dome shape. Tooth-coloured self-cure acrylic resin is then placed in the areas of the natural teeth in the impression. The impression is reseated and the material allowed to set. Once set, the material is trimmed and polished.

The clinician should aim to retain at least two roots to support an overdenture. The maintenance of these roots is onerous, as covering tooth and gingival tissues with a denture will predispose them to caries and gingival inflammation respectively (Fig 1-5). At the outset of treatment to provide overdentures, the patient should be shown how to clean plaque from the root faces. This can be done using a tufted interdental brush or an electric toothbrush. Further requirements include:
- The use of a fluoride toothpaste.
- The denture should be removed at night time and steeped in a denture cleaner.
- The use of a daily fluoride mouth rinse.
- Professional application of fluoride gels or varnishes.

8

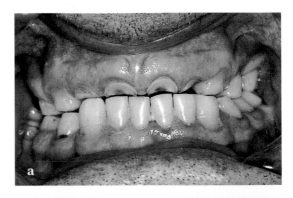

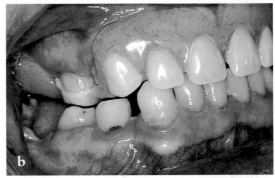

Fig 1-4 (a, b) Removable partial overdenture to restore appearance in a patient with tooth wear.

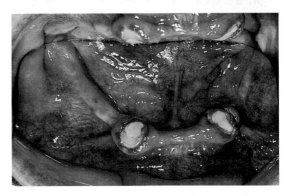

Fig 1-5 Overdenture abutments which have become carious.

The patient should have regular reviews with the dentist and the abutments should be checked carefully for signs of caries and periodontal disease. Even if the patient loses these roots, they will hopefully have learned the complex skills necessary to control complete replacement dentures.

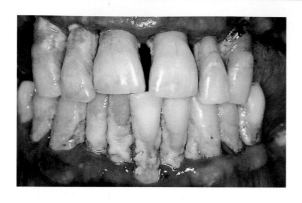

Fig 1-6 Patient with a terminal dentition with poor prognosis due to gross neglect.

Complete **immediate** *replacement dentures*

In some situations, the initial presentation is very unfavourable, and the extent of disease and its consequences is such that the clinician has no option other than to extract the remaining natural teeth without providing a transitional denture. It is unlikely that the patient will accept this without some form of replacement, and the technique of immediate replacement dentures is designed to restore appearance and function at the time of extraction of the remaining teeth. An example of such a case is shown in Fig 1-6. This patient had no regard for his teeth, but had experienced discomfort as many of the teeth had become loose. The prognosis for the remaining natural dentition was very poor and complete immediate denture therapy was planned.

The goals of immediate denture therapy are to maintain satisfactory appearance and function during the post-extraction phase of treatment. The clinical and laboratory stages of providing complete immediate replacement dentures are as follows:

- Discussing the consequences of tooth loss with the patient and explaining clearly the treatment plan. The patient must understand that the tissues will change during the healing period following dental extractions and that frequent adjustment of the dentures may be required. The patient must also be advised that immediate dentures are intended to be temporary, and will probably have to be replaced after 6–12 months. Prior to proceeding with this treatment option, as with any interventive procedure, consent must be secured prior to commencing treatment.
- Recording impressions of the teeth in irreversible hydrocolloid in a stock tray. Construct a customised impression tray and record a working impression in irreversible hydrocolloid.
- Recording the jaw relationship using an interocclusal record, or, in the

presence of large saddle areas, wax record rims. Select teeth of appropriate shade and mould.

- Setting up teeth in the saddle areas in wax and confirming balanced articulation in the mouth. Measure the periodontal pockets around the anterior natural teeth and record the measurements on the laboratory prescription sheet.
- In the dental laboratory, the technician prepares the cast by removing the anterior teeth and scribing the cast using the periodontal pocket depth measures as a guide. Teeth are waxed onto the cast and the dentures are flasked, packed and processed.
- The finished complete dentures are returned to the clinic. The clinician extracts the remaining natural teeth and inserts the complete immediate dentures.
- The patient is instructed to leave the dentures in situ for the next 24 hours. An appointment is arranged for the following day to inspect the dentures and tissues, and to make minor adjustments.
- The patient is advised to take the dentures out only for cleaning but to continue full time wear for a further week.
- At one-week review, further adjustments to occlusion and extensions may be required.
- Review at one month. Adjust as necessary. A chairside reline using a resilient or hard liner may be required at this stage or during the next six months.
- After six months, a definitive treatment plan is made. Options at this stage would be to provide new replacement dentures or to rebase the immediate replacement dentures.

Key Clinical Points

- Avoid loss of remaining natural dentition in old age if at all possible.
- Long-term strategy for preservation of roots to support an overdenture at the very least.
- Transitional removable partial dentures are a valuable aid when further tooth loss is inevitable.
- In an edentate maxilla, stability of a maxillary complete denture may be increased by increasing the number of posterior contacts with the mandible. This can be achieved with either fixed or removable prostheses.

Conclusions

- There has been a shift in the timing of total tooth loss, and many older adults are likely to lose their natural teeth late in life.
- There are a number of techniques available which may increase the possibility of an older adult adapting to complete replacement dentures.
- Long-term treatment planning is essential to avoid the potential consequences of tooth loss late in life.
- Good communication with the patient is necessary. They should understand at an early stage their role in maintaining as many of their natural teeth as possible.

Chapter 2
Assessment of the Edentulous Patient

Aim

The aim of this chapter is to outline the procedures for assessing edentulous patients.

Outcome

At the end of the chapter, the practitioner should understand that there are many functional and psychological consequences of edentulousness. These are difficult to rectify with complete replacement dentures, and a successful outcome depends on clinical and patient-related factors. The practitioner should realise that a treatment plan should take into account these factors, and that the plan should be tailored to the needs of the individual. This includes preliminary treatment designed to improve the health of the denture-bearing area. It should be recognised that good clinical technique is important in preserving healthy tissue and function.

Consequences of Edentulousness

The *anatomical* changes which occur following extraction of natural teeth can broadly be divided into intraoral and extraoral changes. These will differ between individuals who remain partially dentate and those who become edentulous. As people age, loss of alveolar bone is inevitable. However, following total tooth loss, alveolar bone resorption is greatly increased. Alveolar bone height and width decreases markedly (Figs 2-1, 2-2). Most of this change occurs in the first year following extraction, but remains an inexorable process throughout life. Resorption occurs on the buccal aspect of the maxillary ridge and the lingual aspect of the mandibular ridge. Despite extensive research, the reason for the great individual variation in bone loss remains unclear. It seems likely that a combination of local and systemic factors may be responsible for this phenomenon.

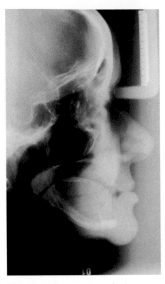

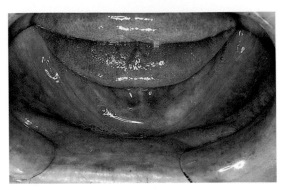

Fig 2-2 Edentulous mandible with gross alveolar resorption.

Fig 2-1 Lateral cephalogram of a 62-year-old patient with severe alveolar resorption.

Further consequences of tooth loss include:
- impaired mastication
- limitation of food selection, especially nutritious foods such as fruits and vegetables
- speech impairment
- change in appearance
- psychosocial impact.

The influence of tooth loss on *masticatory ability*, *masticatory performance* and *dietary selection* has been well documented. Objective tests of masticatory performance indicate that chewing efficiency of edentulous adults is approximately 20% that of dentate individuals. Subjective tests which assess patients' attitudes to food choice suggest that edentulous patients tend to favour highly flavoured soft foods which are of low nutritional value. Reasons for this are complex, and include socioeconomic factors as well as denture-related causes. Surveys of nutritional intake report that edentulous adults have a lower intake of fibre, vitamin C and other important nutrients compared with dentate adults. This suggests that edentulous patients with poor quality diet are at a higher risk of serious illness, including cardiovascular disease and cancer.

Loss of anterior teeth affects *speech* and can be a difficult problem to deal with, particularly in patients with a skeletal Class 2 jaw relationship. In addition to preserving bone, teeth support soft tissues such as the cheeks and lips. These, in turn, influence *appearance*, which is adversely affected once teeth are lost. This is most noticeable in the circumoral region, as the commisures of the lips collapse inwards. A further consequence is loss of vertical dimension and this has the effect of approximating the chin to the nose (Fig 2-3). Some of these changes can be rectified by complete replacement dentures, but there are some limitations. In cases of severe resorption, it may be impossible to meet the patient's aesthetic requirements and, at the same time, provide stable replacement dentures.

Increasingly, researchers are beginning to look at wider issues of health-related *quality of life*. As well as effect on function, it is now recognised that tooth loss has much broader social

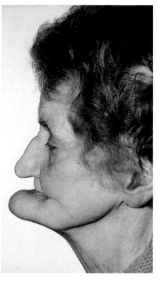

Fig 2-3 Edentulous patient without dentures. Note the approximation of the chin to the nose.

and psychological impact. Acceptance of tooth loss and complete replacement dentures is variable and subjective. Research indicates that patients who have lost their natural teeth have poorer oral health-related quality of life than patients with their own teeth. From a clinical point of view, the outcome of complete replacement dentures in the rehabilitation of edentulousness is difficult to predict. As described above, there are a number of difficult functional problems to overcome. Still, some patients manage very well with technically inadequate dentures. It would appear that satisfaction with the outcome is not always strongly correlated with the technical quality of dentures or the denture-bearing tissues. Some studies also indicate that patients with denture-wearing difficulties score highly on neuroticism indices. Whilst complete replacement dentures continue to be successful for many patients, there are significant numbers of edentulous patients for whom these dentures will not be satisfactory. Despite this, there is ample evidence that well-constructed complete dentures help provide satisfactory oral health-related quality of life for many edentulous patients.

Planning New Complete Dentures

The aim of the first visit is to assess the patient and to formulate a treatment plan. The treatment plan should address the specific requirements of the individual patient. Care should be taken not to leap into the clinical phase of treatment without carefully listening to the patient's complaint. There is wide variation in patient satisfaction with the outcome of complete denture therapy, and the ability of the patient to adapt to change and to the limitations of complete denture therapy should be assessed. It is at this stage that patient expectations should also be determined.

The dental practitioner will encounter a wide variety of presentations, such as: patients with very old dentures and poor quality denture-bearing areas; very old, frail patients; "maladaptive" patients; and patients unhappy with, and seeking, replacement of new dentures.

Assessment of the Patient

The patient's concerns regarding their current dentures and their aspirations for treatment must be assessed. The patient should be asked about the following:

- Reason for replacing dentures.
- Is this problem longstanding or of recent onset?
- How long have they been edentulous?
- How many sets of complete dentures have they had in the past?
- Medical history.
- Social history.

Perhaps the most common problem is that of "loose" dentures. This may be the only complaint, or it may be one of a number of complaints, including:

- pain
- dissatisfaction with appearance
- inability to chew food
- speech problems
- damaged acrylic or fracture of a denture.

Many patients are able to articulate the precise problem they have with their dentures. However, some patients find it difficult to express the nature of their problem, and the clinician should devote some time to eliciting the complaint in such cases. The clinician should enquire about the duration of the complaint. Once the nature of the complaint has been determined, the next stage is to relate this complaint to the examination findings.

Details of the patient's medical history should be recorded. This can be done using a self-completion proforma, but should be carefully checked by the clinician when assessing the patient. Of particular relevance in treating edentulous patients are factors likely to influence adaptation to wearing dentures and factors affecting tolerance of the treatment process. These include:

- Neuromuscular disorders, e.g. Parkinson's disease; stroke
- Dry mouth (xerostomia) associated with
  - medications, e.g. antihypertensives, diuretics, antidepressants
  - diabetes mellitus
  - salivary gland disease
  - post radiotherapy to the orofacial region
- Psychiatric illness
- Nutritional deficiency (may be associated with burning mouth syndrome)
- Arthritis (affects the treatment process).

The patient's social history should also be discussed. If they smoke and/or consume alcohol, the clinician should enquire about the amount and frequency, bearing in mind that these are aetiological factors in the development of oral cancer. If the patient lives at a considerable distance from the surgery, can they attend for the number of visits required to make dentures? If they rely on a relative or friend to bring them to the surgery, will they be able to come for each and every visit?

Examination of the Patient

Following assessment of the patient, a thorough clinical examination should be undertaken, including:

- extraoral examination
- intraoral examination
- dentures in situ
- dentures out of the mouth.

Extraoral examination

At the outset, one should assess the "biological" age of the patient in relation to the chronological age, as this is a useful prognostic indicator. The patient shown in Fig 2-4 is 91 years old and lives independently. He has been edentulous for 60 years and has learned to adapt to dentures extremely well. He has an active social life, and the prognosis for treatment is considered good. In contrast, the patient shown in Fig 2-5 is 53 years old and has poor general health. He appears much older than his chronological age, and may struggle to cope with new complete dentures.

17

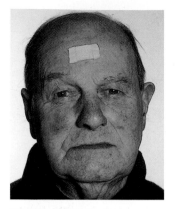

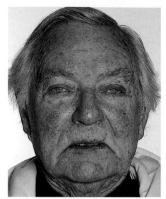

Fig 2-4 Biological versus chronological age – 91-year-old edentulous, independently living male.

Fig 2-5 Biological versus chronological age – 53-year-old male with poor health.

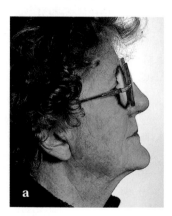

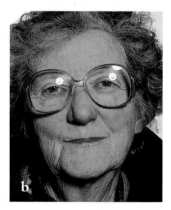

Fig 2-6 Edentulous patient with dentures in place: (a) lateral view (b) facial view.

In the facial region, the patient's skeletal profile should be assessed with the dentures in situ (i.e. Class 1, 2 or 3) bearing in mind that, following loss of the occluding vertical dimension due to wear of the denture teeth, the mandible may appear prognathic (Fig 2-6). Take note of the muscle tone and assess lip support and the proximity of the chin to the nose in both facial and lateral views (Fig 2-6). If the patient has a neuromuscular disorder or has had a cerebrovascular accident (stroke), muscle tone should be carefully noted.

The health of the tissues, particularly the lips and corners of the mouth, should also be assessed and any pathology diagnosed and treated.

Intraoral examination
The following aspects are of particular interest in the intraoral examination:
- The condition of the denture-bearing tissues. This includes the height of the residual alveolar ridge, the condition of the supporting tissues and the presence of mucosal lesions and non-pathological conditions such as bony exostoses.
- The condition of the dentures themselves.

Ridge dimensions
The height and width of the alveolar ridge should be assessed. Shallow ridges offer little stability, and they may have resorbed to the extent that the genial tubercles and mylohyoid ridge become superficial. If the ridge is narrow, then it may not provide adequate support for a denture. The presence of bony exostoses ("tori") should be noted. These are most commonly seen in the centre of the palate and on the lingual aspect of the anterior mandible. If they are prominent, then it may be impossible to extend the denture into the sulcus and this will affect denture retention. In this situation, prominent tori may need to be surgically removed.

Soft tissues
The tissues overlying the ridges should be examined visually and palpated. Ideally, the tissues should be firm and healthy (Fig 2-7). When the tissues are not healthy, retention and stability of the dentures may be compromised. If the tissues are inflamed, then the cause of the inflammation should be determined. Common causes of inflammation of the oral tissues are trauma and candidal infection. Oral manifestations of blood dyscrasias (e.g. iron-deficiency anaemia, leukaemia) may also be present. If salivary flow has diminished, the mucosa will feel dry and this will affect comfort and denture retention. Areas of thin mucosa offer poor support for a denture and may not be resistant to trauma. Management strategies for this situation are discussed in Chapter 7. Areas of mobile, flabby tissue should be noted, as these will compromise retention and stability. The presence of pathological conditions should also be checked. Common pathological conditions associated with denture-wearing include chronic candidal infection and denture-induced hyperplasia. The clinician should also bear in mind the possibility of neoplasia. This may be associated with chronic irritation due to overextended areas of a denture (Fig 2-8).

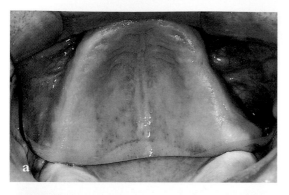

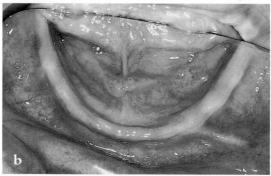

Fig 2-7 Healthy ridges free of pathology:(a) maxilla and (b) mandible.

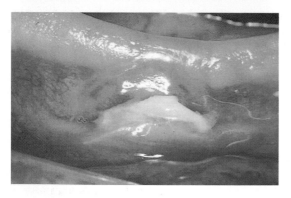

Fig 2-8 Squamous cell carcinoma associated with the overextended periphery of a complete denture.

Dentures in situ

The dentures to be replaced should be inspected in situ, and the retention, stability and support should be assessed. Further features that should be checked include:

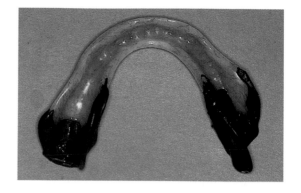

Fig 2-9 Underextended, unstable mandibular complete denture. Green stick tracing compound has been added to extend denture over the retromolar pads prior to rebasing.

- adaptation of the bases to the underlying tissues
- positioning of the denture periphery relative to the sulcus and extension over the retromolar pads (lower denture) and tuberosities (upper denture)
- positioning of the postdam
- positioning of the teeth relative to the muscles of the lips, cheeks, tongue and the floor of mouth
- whether the centric relation coincides with the position of maximum intercuspation of the teeth
- the occluding vertical dimension and freeway space.

The *adaptation* of the dentures to the underlying tissues can be checked by applying gentle finger pressure to both sides of the denture and rotating it. If the denture moves noticeably, then it is poorly adapted. This indicates that the denture is unstable and that there is poor resistance to horizontal forces.

Ideally, the periphery of a complete denture should have intimate contact with the sulcus and should not be displaced during functional movements. The *peripheral extensions* of the dentures should be checked and areas of over- and underextension identified. If there is a space between the denture periphery and the sulcus on gentle manipulation of the tissues, then the periphery is underextended. When the periphery is overextended, the denture is easily displaced and in some cases, overextension is associated with areas of soreness in the sulcus. A common finding is that the lower denture base does not extend over the retromolar pads (Fig 2-9), and there is poor resistance to anteroposterior movement.

The *positioning of the postdam* should be noted by asking the patient to say "aah". This will identify the vibrating line and indicate whether the posterior extension of the maxillary denture is correctly positioned. The best position for a postdam is on the junction of the hard and soft palate as indicated by the vibrating line. Anatomically, this tissue is compressible and is part of the attached soft palate.

The *positioning of the teeth* relative to the surrounding musculature can be checked by gently manipulating the muscles of the lips and cheeks and then visualising contact with the teeth and polished surfaces of the denture. If there is very little contact then there is scope to move the teeth to improve the prospect of achieving a facial seal. Conversely, if the denture is displaced by the tissues during gentle movement, then this should be rectified by altering the position of the teeth and placing them in a position of minimal conflict with the tissues (also known as the *neutral zone*).

The *occlusal relationship* is assessed by asking the patient to close slowly on their posterior teeth. If the patient has developed a posturing habit, then they should be guided gently into centric relation (definition given in Chapter 4). It is helpful to describe to the patient what you are trying to achieve, and the procedure may need to be repeated until a consistent relationship is reproduced. Ideally, there should be even contact without sliding movements in centric relation. It is unlikely, however, that centric relation will coincide with maximum intercuspation with the old dentures and the nature and magnitude of any discrepancy should be noted.

Finally, the *amount of freeway space* should be assessed, and a variety of instruments and techniques are available for this purpose. Freeway space is the difference between the vertical dimension when the muscles are at rest and the occluding vertical dimension, as illustrated in Fig 2-10. The amount of freeway space can be assessed visually by asking the patient to close their teeth together and looking at them from the front and the side. In this way, the clinician can judge whether the patient is overclosed (too much freeway space), propped open (too little freeway space) or they have an appropriate amount of freeway space (Fig 2-11). The amount of freeway space can then be measured by using a Willis bite gauge or by the dot and divider technique (illustrated in Chapter 4). This task often yields highly variable results and the clinician should use the information only to confirm their impression from the clinical assessment. In the authors' experience, the following precautions decrease the variability in measurements:

- The patient should be seated in a comfortable, upright position with their head fully supported by the headrest.
- The resting vertical dimension should be measured with the dentures in

vertical dimension at rest   occluding vertical dimension

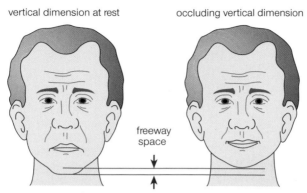

freeway space

Fig 2-10 Determination of freeway space.

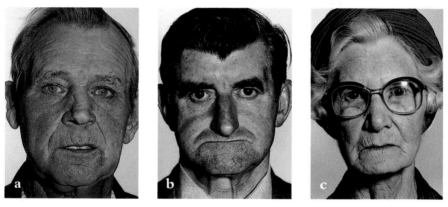

Fig 2-11 Assessment of occluding vertical dimension and freeway space. A patient with (a) too little freeway space; (b) too much freeway space; (c) correct freeway space.

situ – if the teeth contact when measuring resting vertical dimension, then the jaw muscles are not at rest.
- If using the Willis bite gauge method, ensure that the angulation of the instrument is the same when measuring the resting and occluding vertical dimensions.
- When using the dot and dividers technique, ensure that the skin overlying the chin does not move when recording the measurements.

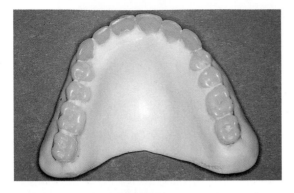

Fig 2-12 Complete denture which has a bleached appearance due to inappropriate cleaning technique. The patient regularly immersed the denture in boiling water.

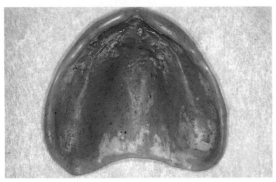

Fig 2-13 Poor denture hygiene. Note the plaque deposits on the fitting surface of the denture.

Dentures – external assessment

The condition of the dentures should be assessed out of the mouth. The clinician should examine the bases for evidence of repairs or abnormal wear and tear. If the denture has been repaired, the patient should be asked when this occured and how did the denture fracture in the first place. Common causes of denture fracture during wearing include flexing of the maxillary denture around a midline torus or prominent incisive papilla, a poorly adapted denture and excessive relief of the maxillary labial fraenum. Denture fracture may also occur if the patient has parafunctional habits or if the maxillary denture is opposed by a natural dentition. If any of these features are implicated in the aetiology of the denture fracture, then the treatment plan should include a strategy for dealing with the problem. This will be discussed in greater detail in later chapters. If the dentures have a bleached appearance or show signs of abrasion (Fig 2-12), then this would indicate an inappropriate cleaning technique. Alternatively, the dentures may be covered in plaque and food material (Fig 2-13) and indicate that the patient does not clean the dentures. In either case, denture cleaning advice would be appropriate.

Formulation of the Treatment Plan

After taking a thorough history and assessing the patient's existing dentures, the clinician should turn their attention to the formulation of a treatment plan. This should, of course, be directed towards solving the patient's presenting complaint. The prognosis for the treatment should be assessed and depends on factors related to the condition of the denture-bearing areas, the attitude of the patient and the ability of the patient to adapt to change. The clinician should recognise that "maladaptive" patients include those who fail to adapt emotionally and those whose failure to adapt to edentulousness is caused by physical limitations. It is vital to discuss with the patient the changes that are feasible at this stage – good communication increases the chances of a successful outcome. If expectations are unrealistic, then this must be addressed prior to construction of new dentures. The treatment plan for new complete replacement dentures should include planning for:

- The impression surface.
- The polished surface and the positioning of teeth in relation to the oral and facial musculature.
- The shape, shade and arrangement of teeth.
- The occlusal surface.

As a consequence of alveolar resorption, the impression surfaces of old dentures will usually be poorly adapted to the underlying tissues. The periphery of the dentures may also be under- or overextended. The clinician should identify these areas and aim to correct them in the new dentures.

The polished surfaces of the dentures are important from functional and aesthetic perspectives. The flanges of the dentures should fill the vestibule to enhance the prospect of achieving a peripheral seal. Regarding tooth position, the inclination of the teeth and their buccolingual position should be considered. Lip support is dependent on the position of the teeth and not the thickness of the denture flange (Fig 2-14). This can be improved by changing the inclination of the teeth and can be demonstrated to the patient by adding wax to the labial aspect of the maxillary teeth on their existing denture.

In terms of occlusion, the clinician must decide if a change in occluding vertical dimension is indicated. This depends on the appearance of the teeth,

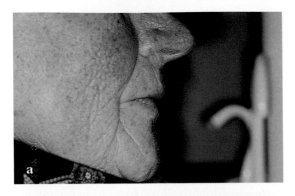

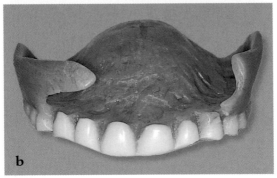

Fig 2-14 Influence of tooth position on lip support. (a) The patient has had the same dentures for 49 years. (b) Satisfactory lip support has been achieved by good tooth position, not the flange.

the facial musculature, phonetics and chewing efficiency. If the patient is overclosed, they are likely to complain of poor appearance and reduced chewing efficiency. The freeway space should be reduced by increasing the occluding vertical dimension and the treatment plan must indicate how this is to be achieved. If the vertical dimension is increased by more than 5 mm, then the patient may not tolerate this change. The change can be assessed gradually using occlusal pivots as discussed later. An increase in occluding vertical dimension can be achieved by raising the occlusal plane of the mandibular denture, dropping the occlusal plane of the maxillary denture or a combination of both. It should be remembered that raising the occlusal plane of the mandibular denture may compromise stability. When there is insufficient freeway space, there is usually discomfort over the mandibular denture-bearing area and in the facial musculature. This tends to get worse through the day. Speech is usually affected. In this situation, the freeway space should be increased by lowering the mandibular occlusal plane or raising the maxillary occlusal plane or both. The choice here is dependent on aesthetic requirements.

Once a treatment plan has been formulated, the goals of this plan should be carefully discussed with the patient. An essential element in achieving a successful outcome is *communication*. Failure to include the patient's wishes in the treatment plan is likely to compromise success. Some of these wishes may be unrealistic and it is important that clinician and patient work together towards a common goal.

Preliminary Treatment

Two aspects of preliminary treatment are considered here:
• The condition of the soft tissues and the underlying bony ridge.
• The condition of the pretreatment complete dentures.

It is prudent to take a panoramic radiograph of the tissues prior to constructing complete replacement dentures. This may reveal the presence of asymptomatic pathology such as retained roots or residual radicular cysts. If the radiograph shows the presence of pathology, then this should be treated prior to making new dentures. In some cases, no treatment is indicated but the patient should be informed of the presence of an anomaly on their radiograph.

Preliminary treatment – treating pathology
Candidal infection
Chronic candidal infection affects the denture-bearing area of the maxilla and has a variety of presentations (Fig 2-15). It has a multi-factorial aetiology and is associated with poor denture hygiene (Fig 2-16), tissue trauma from an ill-fitting denture, constant wearing of the denture and dry mouth. A further manifestation of candidal infection, angular chelitis (Fig 2-17), can be seen at the corners of the mouth and is associated with excessive freeway space and poor denture hygiene. Patients with this condition usually have a diet with a high carbohydrate content. From a denture-wearing perspective, this condition should ideally be resolved prior to making new dentures. Failure to resolve the inflammation in the palate is likely to lead to a poorly adapted denture and thus poor retention. The patient should be instructed to leave their dentures out at night time, soaked in a denture-cleaning agent (e.g. alkaline peroxidase or sodium hypochlorite). Patients may sometimes be unhappy to comply with this advice and the rationale for removing the dentures at night should be carefully explained. Instructions on how the dentures should be cleaned should also be given, especially when the patient

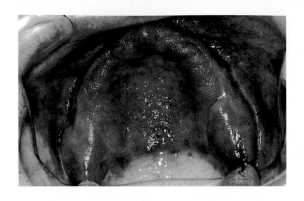

Fig 2-15 Chronic candidal infection affecting the denture-bearing area in an edentulous patient.

refuses to remove the dentures at night. In some cases, there will be evidence of denture-cleaning procedures which are damaging to the dentures, including the use of abrasive agents or soaking the dentures in boiling water. In addition to cleaning instructions it may be appropriate, at this stage, to address the issue of trauma to the tissues from the existing dentures. Usually, this is caused by poor adaptation or physical deterioration of the impression surface of the denture. Tissue conditioners such as Viscogel™ can be used to improve the fit of dentures in the short term. The technique for applying these resilient materials involves the following steps:

1. Following thorough cleaning, trim the periphery of the denture by approximately 2 mm, and apply an adhesive agent (supplied with the tissue conditioner kit) to the entire periphery and fitting surface of the denture.
2. Mix the tissue conditioner according to the manufacturer's instructions and apply evenly over the entire fitting surface of the denture.
3. Seat the denture in the patient's mouth and get them to gently close their teeth together. Perform muscle trimming movements to record the functional sulcus and allow the material to set.
4. Remove from the mouth and trim away any excess material using a warmed scalpel blade. These materials are resilient, so they will feel soft to touch.
5. Allow one to two weeks for the inflammation to resolve. The material will start to degenerate after three weeks, and this may cause trauma to the tissues.
6. If the inflammation does not fully resolve, then a second application of tissue conditioner may be indicated.

If the patient complies with the cleaning instructions and the advice to leave the dentures out at night, then the inflammation should resolve. Occasion-

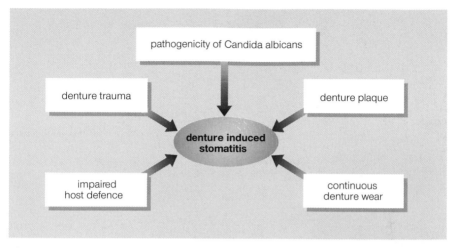

Fig 2-16 Aetiological factors associated with chronic candidal infection in the mouth.

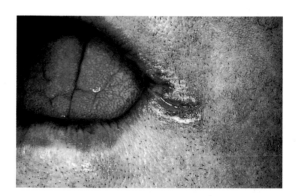

Fig 2-17 Angular chelitis in a patient with chronic candidal infection.

ally, it is appropriate to prescribe an antifungal agent but these should not be considered as first-line treatment. Topical antifungal agents can be applied to the denture in the form of an ointment (miconazole [Daktarin™]) or as pastilles (amphotericin [Nystatin™]). If the condition still shows no sign of abating despite removal of trauma and patient compliance, then referral of the patient for specialist advice may be warranted.

Denture hyperplasia
This is also known as denture granuloma, and is caused by chronic irritation of the mucosa, usually by an overextended denture (Fig 2-18). Some lesions

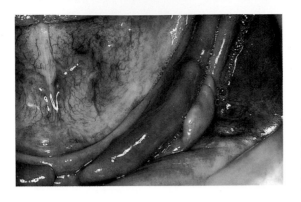

Fig 2-18 Denture-induced granuloma in the buccal sulcus associated with an overextended denture periphery.

are very small indeed, and may not cause immediate problems for denture construction. Longstanding lesions usually present as circumscribed mass of tissue of varying size. The patient should be encouraged to leave the denture out of the mouth as much as possible for six to eight weeks, and the clinician should radically relieve the area of overextension associated with the lesion. Small lesions will usually resolve within two months. Large lesions may not resolve completely, and may have to be removed surgically. This should be undertaken with care, as surgical removal will lead to scar tissue and may further compromise the retention of the denture. The clinician should also be vigilant for potential neoplastic changes in these lesions and consider sending a biopsy of the lesion for a pathological examination if unsure of the diagnosis. If neoplasia is confirmed, then the patient must be referred urgently to a maxillofacial surgeon for treatment.

Preliminary treatment – improving the denture-bearing area

Occasionally, the clinician is presented with a potentially unfavourable denture-bearing area. This may be due to replacement of the bony ridge with fibrous tissue, high frenal attachments or bony prominences. These conditions can be managed using surgical or non-surgical techniques, and the choice depends on the severity of the underlying problem. The non-surgical approach is more commonly used, and impression techniques used to address unfavourable denture-bearing tissues are described in detail in Chapter 3. Disadvantages of surgery include significant morbidity and scarring which further compromises denture retention.

"Flabby ridge"

Excessive fibrous tissue can be displaced during function leading to poor stability and retention of the denture. This condition, commonly known as

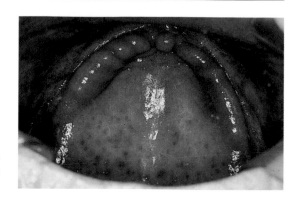

Fig 2-19 Fibrous replacement ("flabby ridge") of the anterior maxillary ridge.

"flabby ridge" (Fig 2-19), is frequently seen in the anterior maxilla and is believed to be due to trauma from the anterior mandibular teeth when missing posterior teeth have not been replaced with a removable partial denture. The mobility of the tissue can be assessed using a ball-ended instrument. When fibrous replacement occurs in the posterior maxilla, there may be insufficient inter-ridge space to place complete upper and lower dentures. Preprosthetic surgery may be indicated in this situation, particularly if the fibrous tissue has proliferated to the extent that the inter-ridge space is significantly reduced. The problem of the flabby ridge may be overcome using a suitable impression technique and this is described in greater detail in Chapter 3.

High frenal attachments
In a case of high frenal attachments, there may have been a persistent problem with denture retention. Usually, the patient will report that the denture dislodges without warning during a functional movement such as smiling or whilst talking. On examination, if the denture fits well and is not overextended, then the cause of the problem may be high frenal attachments on the residual bony ridge (Fig 2-20). Using a simple surgical procedure, the clinician can detach the frenal attachments and, using a suitable surgical template, these will reattach to the ridge in a more favourable position. Complete dentures can then be constructed in the usual way. Surgery should only be contemplated if the fraena are attached at or very close to the crest of the residual ridge. Otherwise, careful attention to muscle trimming when recording the functional impression will usually solve the problem.

Bony prominences
Residual ridge resorption can lead to an uneven ridge which offers poor sup-

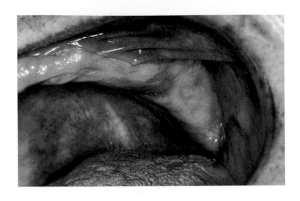

Fig 2-20 High frenal attachments which may affect denture retention.

port for a complete replacement denture (Fig 2-21). In addition, areas such as the genial tubercles and mylohyoid ridge can become exposed. The mucosa overlying these sharp bony prominences can be very thin and not very resistant to trauma. Pain is elicited in these areas by applying digital pressure to the sharp prominences of bone, which also prevent good adaptation of the denture and thus compromise retention. Preprosthetic surgery may be indicated if the prominence is very pronounced or if a non-surgical approach has failed. This involves raising a mucoperiosteal flap following a relieving incision in the sulcus, and then trimming the bony prominences with a bone bur on a water-cooled surgical hand piece. The patient's denture or a surgical plate should be worn to ensure satisfactory healing of the tissues. A potential drawback of this technique is that scar tissue will form in the incision line, and this may compromise denture retention.

Increasing the size of the denture-bearing area
Prior to the advent of endosseous dental implants, a number of surgical techniques were used widely to increase the denture-bearing area, particularly in the mandible. Such forms of preprosthetic surgery are less commonly employed now, as implant-retained prostheses are becoming more popular for overcoming the problems caused by severe alveolar ridge resorption. Nevertheless, preprosthetic surgery still has a place in treating the edentulous patient as implants may be contraindicated or simply beyond the financial means of the patient. Two approaches may be employed:
1. *Vestibuloplasty* – The denture-bearing area is increased by deepening the sulcus. This involves detaching soft tissues and muscle from the bone and reattaching them at a lower level on the jaw. Tissue grafting to cover exposed bone is sometimes required when detached tissues are moved

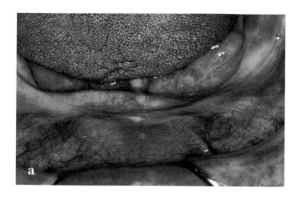

denture trauma

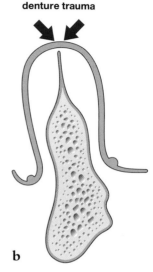

Fig 2-21 Poor primary support for a complete mandibular denture. Note the area of inflammation on the anterior ridge (a) related to prominent bone (b).

b

leaving a defect which would be slow to heal. At least 15 mm of residual alveolus must be available prior to undertaking this procedure.

2. *Ridge augmentation* – The denture-bearing area is enhanced by increasing the height of the bony ridge. Bone harvested from thin bones such as the radius or rib can be shaped to fit the crest of the alveolus. Another approach is to use tissue expanders to increase the space between the mucosa and the underlying bone, and to fill this space after a suitable time with a synthetic material such as hydroxyapatite. A problem with hydroxyapatite is the tendency for the material to become displaced.

These techniques have been used with a measure of success in rehabilitating edentulous patients. However, there are a number of problems associated with them:

- Scar tissue associated with surgery tend to hinder the physical retention of the denture.
- Morbidity associated with preprosthetic surgery, particularly ridge augmentation, is significant.
- Bone grafted onto the residual ridge resorbs quickly, and may disappear completely within two years.
- Synthetic materials are difficult to control, and may penetrate the overlying soft tissues.

Preliminary treatment – diagnostic procedures

Careful treatment planning is essential if the clinician is to achieve a successful outcome with any form of treatment – the construction of complete replacement dentures is no exception. On occasion, there may be some uncertainty about the accuracy of a diagnosis or how well a procedure may be tolerated by the patient. In these circumstances, diagnostic procedures may be undertaken using the existing dentures.

Impression surface

When support for a complete denture is poor, one option is to incorporate a permanent soft lining material in the fitting surface of the denture. These materials do not perform well clinically, and have a lifetime of approximately two years. With such a high maintenance burden, the decision to use these materials should not be taken lightly. The impression surface can be modified with a tissue conditioner to assess how effective a permanent soft lining material is likely to be. The tissue conditioner is added to the fitting surface of the existing denture, and the patient should be reviewed after one to two weeks. If the denture has become comfortable during this period, this is a reasonable predictor of success for a permanent soft lining material.

Occlusal surface

When occlusal surfaces of posterior teeth are very worn, the vertical dimension of occlusion should be raised to improve appearance, function and comfort. However, if the patient has accommodated to a very overclosed position, it may be difficult to record a jaw registration in centric relation, and to assess whether the patient will tolerate a significant increase in occluding vertical dimension. The technique of "occlusal pivots" can be used to gradually increase the occluding vertical dimension. The technique involves the following steps:

1. Add cold-cured acrylic resin to the occlusal surfaces of the lower posterior teeth, and flatten the surface. The thickness of material added to the denture is arbitrary, but around 5 mm should suffice at this stage.
2. Place tin foil over the unset resin, and ask the patient to close until the upper teeth contact the foil. The patient should not be allowed to bite heavily.
3. Allow the material to set, remove the foil, trim and polish.
4. Review the patient after a week and see how well this increase has been tolerated. The clinician can now decide whether to increase or decrease the height of the pivots.
5. When the final occlusal vertical dimension has been determined (Fig 2-22), this information can be incorporated in the new replacement dentures.

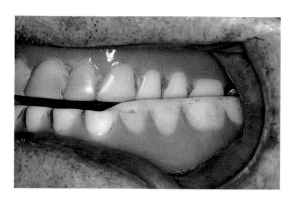

Fig 2-22 Use of acrylic occlusal pivots to assess tolerance of increasing the occlusal vertical dimension in a patient with excessive freeway space.

Tips for Treatment Planning – Summary

- The treatment plan must address the patient's complaints.
- The treatment plan should include a plan for the impression surface, the polished surface and the occlusal surface.
- Substantial changes may need to be introduced gradually to increase the chances of adaptation.
- Ensure that the denture-bearing tissues are healthy prior to denture construction.
- Good communication with the patient is essential.

Conclusions

- The patient's existing dentures should be used for reference when constructing complete replacement dentures.
- The treatment plan should aim to retain and reproduce acceptable features of the old dentures whilst rectifying faults.
- The treatment plan should include a plan for the impression surface, polished surface and occlusal surface.
- Preliminary treatment aimed at improving the health of the denture-bearing areas should be undertaken prior to recording impressions.

Chapter 3
Impression Procedures for Complete Dentures

Aim

The aim of this chapter is to discuss the theory for achieving complete denture retention and the importance of impression procedures.

Outcome

At the end of this chapter, the clinician should understand that creating a retentive denture is reliant on a good understanding of the anatomy of the denture-bearing area, and physical and physiological factors. Recording an impression is a process which requires consideration of the action of the sulcus, the condition of the denture-bearing area, the quality and quantity of saliva and finally the materials used to record the impressions. It must be seen as a two-stage process, with the primary and secondary impression stages having distinct, important functions. If sufficient attention is paid to recording good quality primary and secondary impressions, then the denture should be retentive.

Impression Theory

Retentive complete dentures are reliant on the interplay between forces of retention, stability and support. To describe these succinctly, *retention* depends on forces which resist displacement of the denture away from the denture-bearing area; *stability* relies on resisting forces likely to displace the denture laterally or anteroposteriorly; and *support* is provided by factors which resist displacement of the denture into the denture-bearing tissues. The important relationship between these forces is shown in Fig 3-1. Although this chapter is devoted to a discussion of impression making, the reader should bear in mind that these factors are inter-related. If, for example, one has created a retentive denture but introduced occlusal errors into the occlusal scheme of the dentures, then the resultant instability of the dentures caused by the unbalanced occlusion may overcome the forces designed to retain the denture. Similarly, apparently satisfactory retentive forces can be overcome by an unstable denture-bearing area such as a flabby alveolar ridge.

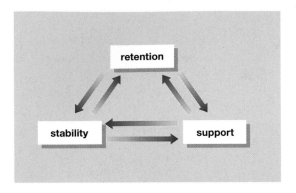

Fig 3-1 Relationship between retention, stability and support. The retention of complete dentures is dependent on the interaction between these forces.

Forces which will make a complete denture retentive have been described as (a) physiological forces and, (b) physical forces.

- *Physiological forces* – These forces are applied to the polished surfaces of the dentures by the muscles of the lips, the cheeks and the tongue. They rely on the patient's ability to learn a complex series of neuromuscular reflexes, and this varies from patient to patient. The patient has to learn to use these muscles to exert retentive forces on the polished surfaces of the dentures during functional movements. Fish described how the clinician should shape the polished surfaces of the dentures to enhance these physiological forces of retention (Fig 3-2). These forces of retention can be harnessed to overcome some of the limitations of complete dentures, and may help explain why patients can control technically inadequate dentures. It is possible that the ability of patients to control dentures diminishes with age, and keeping a familiar polished surface shape may be critical to the outcome of new replacement complete dentures. This is the theoretical basis for the copy denture technique described in Chapter 9.
- *Physical forces* – Forces of adhesion, cohesion and surface tension can be harnessed to improve denture retention. In clinical terms, this involves creating a peripheral seal. Air must be excluded between the fitting surface of the denture and the denture-bearing tissues, and an intact salivary film allowed to form on the impression surface of the denture. If this is achieved, forces of cohesion will act to keep the salivary film intact, whilst forces of adhesion and surface tension will act to attract saliva to the denture and the denture-bearing tissues. These forces will be harnessed only if the denture is placed on *compressible* tissues, and it is therefore important that the clinician identifies these in the mouth. The elastic nature of these tissues allows them to recoil around the periphery of the denture when compressed. The

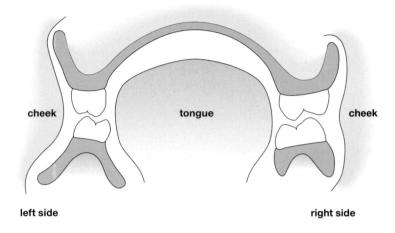

Fig 3-2 Action of muscles on polished surfaces of complete dentures.

compressible areas of soft tissue in the denture-bearing area are the sulci, the attached part of the soft palate and the retromolar pads in the mandible. If the denture is not placed over these areas, then air will escape into the area above the fitting surface and disrupt the layer of saliva. Further factors which influence the physical forces of retention are:

- surface area – the greater the area of coverage, the more retentive the denture will be
- the quantity of saliva – retention decreases as salivary flow diminishes
- the quality of saliva – if saliva is thick with a high mucus content, the dentures are unlikely to be retentive
- the space between the fitting surface of the denture and the denture-bearing area should be as thin as possible.

Anatomy of the Denture-bearing Area:

Two aspects should be considered: (a) gross anatomy of the maxillary and mandibular denture-bearing area; and (b) the histology of the denture-bearing tissues. The retention of complete replacement dentures is influenced by the activity of muscles which define the buccal, labial and lingual sulci, frenal attachments, and the soft palate. These will influence the shape of the periphery of the dentures. Muscle groups also influence the shape of the polished surfaces of the dentures. The muscle groups involved are listed in Table 3-1.

Table 3-1 Muscles which define the maxillary and mandibular denture-bearing areas.

Maxilla	Mandible
Periphery	*Periphery (buccal)*
buccinator	buccinator
levator anguli oris	depressor labii inferioris
incisivus superioris	mentalis
buccal frena	
labial frena	*Periphery (lingual)*
muscles of the soft palate	superior constrictor
	pterygomandibular raphe
	palatoglossus
	mylohyoid
	genioglossus
	lingual frenum
Polished surface shape	*Polished surface shape*
modiolus	anterior border of masseter
	tongue
	modiolus

The anatomy of the denture-bearing area in the *maxilla* is further defined by:
* the residual alveolar ridge
* the root of the zygoma
* the hamular notch
* the maxillary tuberosities
* the attached part of the soft palate.

and in the *mandible* by:
* the residual alveolar ridge
* the external oblique ridge
* the retromolar pads.

The oral mucosa consists of epithelium and connective tissue. It covers the palate and the alveolar ridges, and extends over the muscles of the palate, cheeks and floor of the mouth. In areas where there is friction, the epithelium has the potential to produce keratin which increases resistance to trauma. In certain areas of the mouth, such as the sulci, the oral mucosa is separated from the underlying muscle by a layer of submucosa. This tissue is compressible and suitable for loading with a denture. Areas where the oral mucosa is tightly bound to bone, such as the hard palate, do not have a layer of submucosa and are not compressible. When severe alveolar resorption occurs, prominent spicules of bone such as the genial tubercles can become superficial. The oral mucosa is tightly bound to this bone and offers poor support for a complete denture. These areas should be relieved by placing tin foil on the master cast prior to processing the denture base.

Primary Impressions

The aim of the primary impression is to record the entire denture-bearing area. Failure to record the denture-bearing area on the primary impression will create difficulties in recording a satisfactory definitive impression and ultimately result in a poorly retentive denture. Consequently, it is unwise to disregard the importance of having a satisfactory primary impression in the hope that deficiencies will be rectified in the definitive impression. The nature of primary impressions is such that control of the tissues when recording the impression is minimal, and thus the impression will be overextended. If a denture is made on a model cast from such an impression, then it too will be overextended and not retentive.

Primary impressions should be recorded in rigid stock trays. Examples of edentulous stock trays are shown in Fig 3-3. When recording a primary impression, the clinician should select a tray that most closely fits the denture-bearing area. If the tray is grossly underextended, then green stick tracing compound or beading wax can be added to the tray to improve extension. If the denture-bearing area is particularly small, then overextension of the tray may be a problem. In this situation, a plastic stock tray should be used and areas of overextension can be reduced prior to recording the impression. Impression materials which are commonly used for recording primary impressions are as follows:

- *Irreversible hydrocolloid (alginate)* – This material – alginate – has elastic properties and thus is suitable for recording undercut areas. It must be sup-

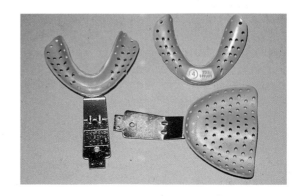

Fig 3-3 Disposable stock trays for use in edentulous patients.

ported by the tray in the areas of the periphery of the denture, or it will not adequately record the sulcus (Fig 3-4). Irreversible hydrocolloid impressions must be cast quickly (ideally within one to two hours of recording the impression), as this is not a dimensionally stable material and is particularly prone to shrinkage. A further concern with the material is that it is difficult to disinfect the impression without distorting the material. Nonetheless, if handled correctly, irreversible hydrocolloid can provide good quality impressions (Fig 3-5).

- *Thermoplastic material (impression compound)* – This material (Fig 3-6) is excellent for recording primary impressions in stock trays as its viscosity ensures that it will flow into the sulcul areas. It should ideally be used in a metal tray, but plastic trays will suffice. It is a rigid material, and therefore will not be suitable for undercut areas. As it is a thermoplastic material (i.e. flows when heated and becomes solid again when cooled) it can be modified. The critical temperature for impression compound is around 54 °C and a thermostatically controlled water bath (Fig 3-7) can be used to keep the material at this temperature. The material is removed from the water bath, kneaded and loaded onto the tray. It is then inserted in the patient's mouth, and the borders moulded and inspected. If unsatisfactory, the material can be softened again, and the impression remade. Minor deficiencies can be addressed by softening the material in the area of the deficiency with a Hanau torch, tempering and reseating the impression.

- *Impression putty* – This is a rigid material and, like impression compound, should ideally be used in a metal stock tray, but a plastic tray will suffice. It is more elastic than compound, and therefore suitable for use in undercut areas. Its main disadvantage is its cost.

Disinfection procedures

Prior to sending impressions to the dental laboratory, they must be disinfected as part of cross-infection control procedures. Dilute 0.5% sodium hypochlorite can be used, but there is evidence that immersion for more than a few minutes diminishes the quality of, in particular, hydrocolloid and polyether impressions. It is recommended that impressions made with these materials be dipped in hypochlorite solution, rinsed and then wrapped in gauze soaked with sodium hypochlorite for ten minutes. A further possibility is to use a disinfection machine. Disinfection procedures should be adhered to for all stages of denture construction including those described in later chapters.

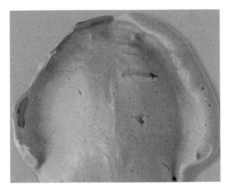

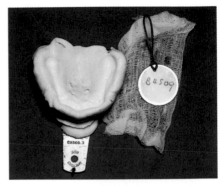

Fig 3-4 Poor quality primary impression with inadequate representation of the sulcus.

Fig 3-5 Good quality alginate impression of the maxillary denture-bearing area.

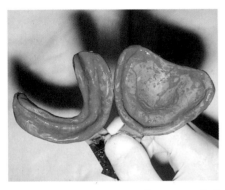

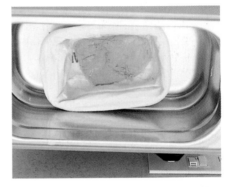

Fig 3-6 Primary impressions recorded in impression compound.

Fig 3-7 Thermostatically controlled water bath used for softening impression compound.

Common Faults With Primary Impressions

1. *Failure to record the entire denture-bearing area.* This occurs when the tray size is inadequate, and the impression material does not reach areas such as the retromolar pad, the full depth of the palate or the distolingual sulcus. The impression tray should be extended to ensure that the impression material reaches these areas, in particular, when using irreversible hydrocolloid impression material.
2. *Insufficient anatomical detail.* The impression material may cover the denture-bearing area, but there is insufficient detail of frenal attachments, or

43

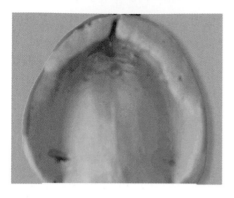

Fig 3-8 Poor quality primary impression with a grossly distorted labial sulcus and inadequate detail of the left posterior sulcus.

the distolingual sulcus. When using a rigid material such as impression compound, this occurs if the material is not soft enough when the impression tray is seated in the mouth. Failure to adequately muscle trim the impression will also lead to insufficient frenal detail. The lingual surface of the mandibular impression should have a sigmoid shape. However, if empty mouth movements, such as swallowing, have not been undertaken during the recording of an impression then the distolingual sulcus will not be adequately recorded.

3. *Impression tray not seated correctly.* This situation arises if the impression tray is rotated or seated incorrectly in an anteroposterior direction (Fig 3-8). In the case of rotation, the sulcus will be grossly distorted on one side and insufficiently recorded on the contralateral side. This will result in a customised tray which is not adequately related to the sulcus and a controlled working impression procedure will not be possible. If the impression tray is seated too far forward, as is often the case in mandibular impressions, then the lingual sulcus and possibly the retromolar areas, will not be adequately recorded.

4. *Distortion of the impression material.* If the impression material is not handled correctly in the dental laboratory, then a poor quality customised impression tray may be the result.

Prescription for Special (Customised Impression) Trays

Once the primary impressions have been satisfactorily recorded, the clinician should prescribe the construction of a customised impression tray. The prescription features of the tray depend on the material that the clinician intends to use to record the definitive working impression. If a mucocompressive technique is used, then a close fitting tray is required, and this should be constructed on the primary model with minimal spacing. If a minimally displacive technique is used, then spacing appropriate for the material is required. Materials which can be used are: (a) irreversible hydrocolloid (3 mm spacing required); (b) impression plaster (2 mm spacing required); and (c) medium or low viscosity elastomers (2 mm spacing required). When using irreversible hydrocolloid, accessory retention for the material can be achieved by perforating the impression tray. In addition to spacing, the clinician should also prescribe the positioning of handles or finger stops on the tray.

Final Impression Techniques

The choice of the final impression technique is dependent on what the clinician is trying to achieve. By using a mucocompressive technique, the aim is to construct the denture on a model of the denture-bearing tissues in a compressed state. A potential difficulty with this approach is that it may increase bone resorption, but there is little evidence to support this theory. The minimally displacive approach aims to compress the tissues in the sulcus but not on the alveolar ridge. In both techniques, it is important that the periphery of the impression records the shape of the functional sulcus, as this will facilitate the development of a peripheral seal.

Whichever technique is chosen, the customised impression tray must be checked on the primary model and in the mouth to see if it is satisfactory. The periphery should be checked for overextension, underextension and adaptation to the denture-bearing area.

In the case of a mucocompressive technique, the steps are as follows:

1. Check the extension of the tray. There should be 2 mm clearance between the sulcus (including the frenal attachments) and the periphery of the tray. Any overextended areas should be trimmed. If the impression tray is grossly underextended, then the tray should be disregarded and a new primary impression made.
2. Identify the vibrating line which defines the attached part of the soft palate by asking the patient to say "aah". The posterior limit of the tray should be trimmed back to just beyond this area.
3. Green stick tracing compound should then be added to the periphery of the tray in a sequential manner and border moulding undertaken. It should also be added to the posterior aspect of the fitting surface of the tray. When the tissues have been compressed, a peripheral seal will develop and the tray should be retentive (Fig 3-9). If it is not retentive, then the green stick is overextended or underextended. When overextended, a peripheral seal develops but is broken when adjacent muscles are moved. If a peripheral seal has not developed, then the green stick has not sufficiently compressed the tissues and more green stick should be added.

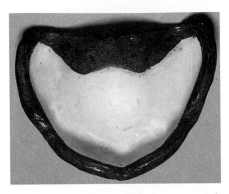

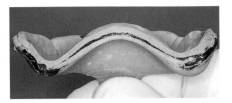

Fig 3-9 Border-moulded green stick tracing compound which had been added to the periphery of the impression tray to achieve a peripheral seal. Note the position of the tracing compound on the posterior aspect of the tray.

Fig 3-10 Mucocompressive impression technique. Note the thin layer of impression paste.

4. When a retentive tray has been prepared satisfactorily, then zinc oxide and eugenol paste should be applied over the fitting surface of the tray and the green stick. The tray should then be reseated, and the borders moulded. Zinc oxide and eugenol paste sets in approximately five minutes, giving a suitable working time.

5. Remove the tray and inspect the impression. If there are any minor deficiencies, these can be filled in with impression wax and the tray reseated in the mouth. This material flows at mouth temperature and suitable for filling minor defects. Large air blows indicate that (a) an insufficient amount of zinc oxide and eugenol paste was added to the tray; or (b) the green stick was not correctly extended; or (c) there was too much space between the fitting surface of the tray and the denture-bearing tissues. Major deficiencies may require a new tray.

6. It is important to trim the impression paste back to the posterior edge of the impression tray. The impression paste should be very thin (Fig 3-10), indicating that the green stick has indeed compressed the tissues. If the paste is thick, then either insufficient green stick has been added or the tray has been seated incorrectly. This can be confirmed by checking the depth of impression material in the anterior part of the tray. If this is thin, or the tray is visible through the impression material, then the tray has been incorrectly seated and a new impression is required.

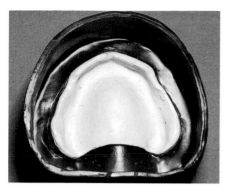

Fig 3-11 Completed maxillary impression which has been beaded with wax to define the denture periphery and then boxed.

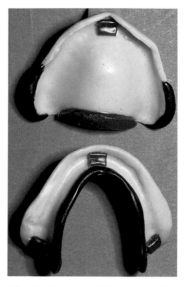

Fig 3-12 Stops added to the fitting surface of impression trays. Note the use of green stick tracing compound to correct underextended areas.

7. Once satisfied with the impression, then it should be beaded and boxed in (Fig 3-11) using beading and carding waxes. This will protect the periphery when the impression is cast by the dental technician.

When using a minimally displacive technique, the steps are as follows:
1. Stops should be visible in the tray if they have been prescribed. If not visible, then stops should be created by adding green stick or wax in three areas of the fitting surface of the tray (Fig 3-12).
2. Areas of overextension of the tray should be trimmed back to allow a sufficient thickness of impression material in the sulcus. Areas of underextension can be altered by adding green stick to improve extension.
3. Impression plaster, irreversible hydrocolloid or elastomer can be used to record the impression. Once loaded with impression material the impression tray should be seated and border moulded.
4. When the material has set, remove the tray and examine the impression. If large air blows are visible, then the impression should be retaken.

5. Once satisfied with the quality of the impression, then it should be beaded and boxed in as described previously. The positioning of the postdam should be indicated to the technician, as the master cast will have to be scribed in this area prior to processing the denture base.

When the final impression has been deemed satisfactory, it should be disinfected prior to being sent to the dental laboratory. The occlusal rims should be prescribed to the technician, and this includes details for the base and the rim. The materials used for the base include self-cured acrylic resin, shellac, wax and heat-cured acrylic resin. Further details of occlusal rim construction will be considered in Chapter 4.

Special Impression Techniques

In some situations, the condition of the denture-bearing area demands the use of special impression techniques. These conditions include:
- Fibrous replacement of the posterior ridge ("unemployed ridge").
- "Flabby ridge" in the anterior maxilla.

Fibrous replacement of the posterior mandibular ridge is evident when clinical examination reveals a mobile band of tissue on the crest of the ridge (Fig 3-13). This arises as a consequence of poor adaptation of the denture to the tissues and results in poor stability and discomfort. A displaceable or flabby anterior maxillary ridge is frequently seen when the edentate maxilla is opposed by natural teeth in the anterior mandible. This combination causes trauma to the anterior maxillary ridge as all occlusal forces are directed onto this area, and fibrous replacement of the bony ridge occurs. This displaceable tissue can result in problems with stability and retention of dentures. Occasionally, fibrous replacement of the posterior maxillary ridge can be seen (Fig 3-14).

The impression techniques described for dealing with these problems are underpinned by the need to avoid displacing mobile tissues when recording the impression. The remainder of the denture-bearing area can be treated as described previously, and hence "selective pressure" techniques have been described for dealing with these clinical situations.

Unemployed ridge
Standard impression techniques, in particular mucocompressive techniques, will displace the mobile band of tissue. A hole should be cut in the customised impression tray in the area corresponding to the fibrous band prior

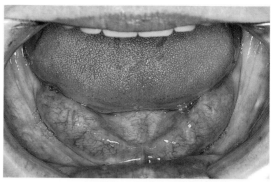

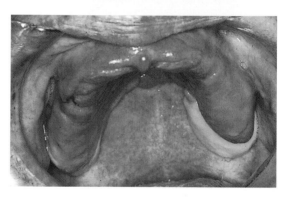

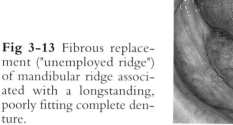

Fig 3-13 Fibrous replacement ("unemployed ridge") of mandibular ridge associated with a longstanding, poorly fitting complete denture.

Fig 3-14 Fibrous replacement of posterior maxillary ridge. This tissue is displaced easily and reduces the interridge space.

to recording the impression with an irreversible hydrocolloid or elastomer. Another approach to this problem is to record an impression of the denture-bearing area using green stick tracing compound in a customised tray. The area of the tray corresponding to the unemployed ridge is perforated and a wash impression in a low viscosity material (e.g. a lightbodied polyvinylsiloxane) is recorded over the entire denture-bearing area.

Flabby maxillary ridge

In this situation the impression technique involves preparing the customised, close fitting tray with a hole over the flabby ridge (Fig 3-15). The technician should be instructed to add finger stops rather than a handle on the tray. The clinical steps are as follows:

1. Check the peripheral extensions of the tray. These should be trimmed so that the periphery is 2 mm short of the functional sulcus. The tray should extend just beyond the vibrating line on the attached part of the soft palate.

49

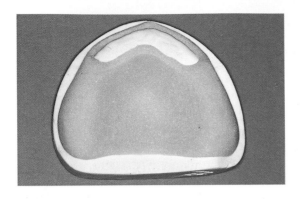

Fig 3-15 Modified impression tray for recording an impression of a flabby ridge.

2. Green stick tracing compound should be added gradually to the periphery of the tray until the functional sulcus is recorded.
3. Apply zinc oxide and eugenol paste to the tray and record an impression. Trim back any impression material which has escaped through the hole in the tray. Check that the remainder of the denture-bearing area has been recorded satisfactorily.
4. Reseat the impression and apply impression plaster over the exposed flabby tissue. This can be applied using a brush or a wax knife. The material should be stiff enough to be applied with a brush, but not runny to the extent that it drips.
5. Remove the impression tray carefully when the impression plaster has set and check that it is satisfactory. Instruct the technician to put a separating agent on the plaster prior to casting the impression.
6. Apply beading wax to the periphery and box the impression.
   Following the same steps, medium and low viscosity polyvinylsiloxane impression materials can be used as alternatives to zinc oxide and eugenol paste and impression plaster respectively.

Tips for Impression Making – Summary

- Be critical of the primary impression. Inadequate primary impressions compromise the process of denture construction.
- The clinician should prescribe special trays and the features required. Do not assume that the dental technician will undertake this task.
- Choose an impression-recording technique and material to suit the tissues you are dealing with.

Conclusions

- A preliminary impression should record the entire denture-bearing area, and inadequate primary impressions may compromise the process of complete denture construction.
- A number of technical and patient–related factors influence denture retention and these should be considered when recording definitive impressions.
- The method and material used should depend on the nature of the denture-bearing area. There are no right and wrong techniques.
- Good quality impressions enhance complete denture retention. Good communication between the dentist and the technician is an essential part of this process.

Reference

Academy of Prosthodontics. Glossary of prosthodontic terms. 7th ed. J Prosthet Dent 1999;81:39-110.

Chapter 4

Registration of the Jaw Relationship

Aim

The aim of this chapter is to describe the stages involved in the recording of the jaw relationship for an edentulous patient.

Outcome

At the end of this chapter, the practitioner should understand the need to prescribe occlusal rim construction with respect to the individual patient's requirements. It should be recognised that the manipulation of occlusal rims to record the jaw relationship and to indicate the desired tooth position must be undertaken in a sequential manner with reference to the treatment plan. The clinician should also understand the rationale for the choice of articulator used to mount working casts for setting up trial denture teeth.

Prescription of Occlusal Rims

Once the working impressions of the patient's denture-bearing area have been made, the clinician should prescribe the construction of occlusal rims. The prescription features should include details of the dimension of the wax rims and the material from which the base should be constructed.

Regarding the rim dimensions, the clinician should refer to the treatment plan. If no major changes are to be made to the vertical height of the existing dentures, then the rims should be of similar vertical and horizontal dimensions. When changes are planned then the size of the rims should reflect these changes and prescribed accordingly. Given an accurate prescription, clinical time will be saved in reducing or building up rims at the chairside.

There are a number of materials available for the construction of the bases:
- self-cured acrylic resin
- heat-cured acrylic resin
- non-precious metal alloy

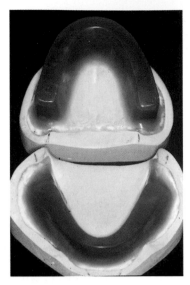

Fig 4-1 Heat-cured acrylic ("permanent") bases.

- wax
- thermoplastic materials (shellac).

Self-cured acrylic resin, wax and thermoplastic materials are considered as "temporary bases" in that they are not incorporated into the final denture. They are easily manipulated and the bases can be constructed quickly. However, these materials are not dimensionally stable, and are poorly adapted to the underlying tissues. This can make them difficult to control in the patient's mouth. Heat-cured bases (Fig 4-1) are considered "permanent bases" as they are ultimately incorporated into the finished denture. When the working impressions have been cast, the base is laid down on the cast. It is then flasked and processed, deflasked and polished. A wax rim is then added to the processed base and it is returned to the clinician on a duplicate model. If the working impressions were satisfactory, the bases should be stable and retentive in the patient's mouth. This, in turn, should make the process of recording the jaw relationship much easier, particularly when there has been significant resorption of the residual alveolar ridge. There are no absolute contraindications to using these bases, but there are some potential disadvantages, such as:

- The base will have to go through a second curing cycle when processing the teeth to the base. In theory, this could cause warpage of the base.
- They consume a greater amount of technical time and therefore are more expensive.
- If there is little inter-ridge space, or if the labial aspect of the anterior maxilla is prominent (i.e. in a skeletal Class 2 case), then room for the wax rim is reduced. In this situation, reduction of the wax rim may leave little wax to retain teeth, and the clinician or technician may have to remove some of the base to add teeth for a trial set-up.
- The working cast is destroyed to make the base.

Metal bases can be made prior to the jaw registration stage, but it is prudent to wait until the trial denture stage has been completed. The rationale for this is that the position of the teeth helps to determine the extent of the base, and therefore an acceptable tooth position should be determined first. They are indicated when there has been a history of denture fracture. However, it should be remembered that they are difficult to adjust and tend to be heavier than acrylic bases. In addition, other alternatives such as high-impact acrylic should also be considered.

Terminology

The terminology used throughout the remainder of this text is that contained in the Glossary of Prosthodontic Terms. In a dentate patient, the position of maximum intercuspation (ICP) or of first contact in a retruded arc of closure – the retruded contact position (RCP) are used to record a jaw relationship. These positions are determined by the natural teeth, which of course are absent in an edentulous patient. When recording a jaw relationship for an edentulous patient, it is desirable to use a reproducible position. There are various terms used for this such as "rest position", "physiologic rest position" and "centric jaw relation". In this text, the term we use is "CENTRIC RELATION" as described by Ash. He defines centric relation as "a maxilla to mandible relationship in which the condyles and the discs are thought to be in the midmost, uppermost position. The position has been difficult to define anatomically but is determined clinically by assessing when the jaw can hinge on a fixed terminal axis (up to 25 mm). It is a clinically determined relationship of the mandible to the maxilla when the condyle–disk assemblies are positioned in their most superior position in the mandibular fossae and against the distal slope of the articular eminence." There are six further definitions of centric relation in the Glossary of Prosthodontic Terms, and this reflects the lack of universal acceptance of any one definition. Our rationale for choosing Ash's definition is that it includes details of how the relationship should be assessed clinically. CENTRIC OCCLUSION is defined as "the occlusion of the opposing teeth when the mandible is in centric relation". Ideally, this should coincide with maximal intercuspation. BALANCED ARTICULATION is defined as "the bilateral, simultaneous, anterior and posterior occlusal contact of teeth in centric and eccentric positions". In this text, as in some other texts, "balanced occlusion" is used to describe the static centric position, whereas "balanced articulation" refers to the dynamic, eccentric position. FREEWAY SPACE is defined as the "difference between the vertical dimension of rest and the vertical dimension while in occlusion". The rest vertical dimension is the "habitual postural jaw relation when the patient is resting comfortably in an upright position and the condyles are in a neutral, unstrained position in the glenoid fossa".

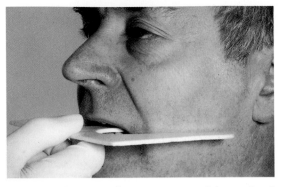

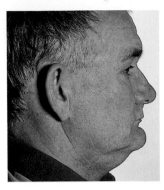

Fig 4-2 Checking the orientation of the occlusal plane with an occlusal plane guide. The rim should be parallel with the alatragal and interpupillary lines. (Courtesy of Mr ID Murray)

Fig 4-3 Assessment of the nasolabial angle which should be approximately 90° with the occlusal rim in situ.

Technique

The jaw registration procedure should be undertaken in a sequential manner with reference to the treatment plan. The rims must be adjusted to meet the requirements for the appearance and the occlusion of the new dentures. The retention and stability of the rims should be checked. If the rims lack retention and are unstable then new impressions may be required. If the occlusal rims are satisfactory, then the maxillary rim should be adjusted first. The aspects of the maxillary rim which must be adjusted are:

- The level of the rim – If the patient was happy with the amount of tooth visible, then the level of the wax rim should be trimmed to this height.
- The orientation of the rim – External landmarks include the interpupillary and the alatragal lines. The rim should be trimmed until its orientation is parallel to these lines. This should be assessed visually, and can be confirmed using a Foxes occlusal plane guide (Fig 4-2).
- The labial profile – The reference point used is the nasolabial angle, and this should be approximately 90° (Fig 4-3).
- The shape of the arch of the rim – This should be trimmed to allow the mucosa of the cheek to lie gently against it and the rim should not be displaced by cheek movement.

Once the maxillary rim has been trimmed, then the mandibular rim should be adjusted. The labial and lingual aspects of the rim should be adjusted until

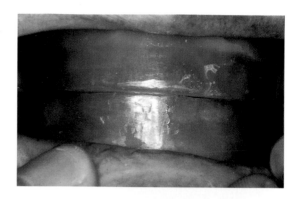

Fig 4-4 Occlusal rims meeting evenly in centric relation at planned OVD.

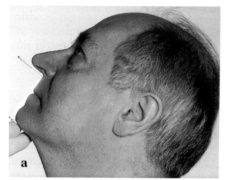
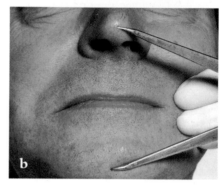

Fig 4-5 Measurement of the OVD using (a) Willis bite gauge and (b) dividers. (Courtesy of Mr ID Murray)

the rim is stable during movements of the lip, tongue and cheek musculature. The occlusal aspect of the rim should then be adjusted until it meets the maxillary rim at the planned occlusal vertical dimension (OVD) (Fig 4-4). The amount of freeway space can be checked using a Willis gauge or dividers (Fig 4-5). Care should be taken that the posterior aspects of the rims ("heels") are not in contact, particularly when permanent bases are used. If they are in contact, then adjustments should be made to take them out of contact prior to further occlusal adjustment.

When adjustments have been completed, then the rims must be sealed together. A number of techniques have been described for this purpose, and the method used is largely one of preference. Materials which can be used to join the rims include wax, silicone and zinc oxide and eugenol paste. What is essential is that the rims can be reassembled accurately outside the mouth in the event that they become separated. Score marks should be placed on the rims on the labial and buccal aspects, starting on the maxillary rim and continuing onto the mandibular rim. The labial mark should correspond to the centre of the face and this can be used to check for lateral errors during the registration process. The buccal score marks can be used to check for protrusive errors.

In patients with a skeletal Class 2 or Class 3 profile, there should be horizontal overlap and the clinician should avoid trimming the rims in an attempt to provide the patient with dentures in a Class 1 relationship.

Choosing an Articulator for Complete Denture Construction

The rims must be articulated to allow the technician to set up teeth for a trial denture. An articulator is defined in the Glossary of Prosthodontic Terms as "a mechanical instrument that represents the temporomandibular joints and jaws, to which maxillary and mandibular casts may be attached to simulate some or all mandibular movements". There are four classes of articulator: (a) the hinge articulator, which allows vertical but not horizontal movement; (b) an articulator which allows horizontal as well as vertical movements but which is not oriented to the temporomandibular joints (e.g. free plane articulator); (c) a semi-adjustable articulator which allows horizontal and vertical movements and simulates condylar pathways by using average values or mechanical equivalents for all part of the motion; and (d) a fully adjustable articulator which can accept three-dimensional dynamic registrations and therefore orientate the casts to the temporomandibular joints and simulate mandibular movements.

Examples of simple hinge and semi-adjustable articulators are shown in Fig 4-6.

As a general rule, as the articulator used increases in sophistication, the amount of chairside adjustment of the occlusal surfaces diminishes. When deciding which articulator to use, the clinician must ask "What are you trying to achieve?" If the aim of treatment is to use anatomical teeth to achieve balanced articulation, then a semi-adjustable articulator should be used. In some edentulous cases, the pretreatment examination will reveal an unusual pattern of wear on the denture surfaces. This could indicate a chewing pattern similar to a dentate patient, and the use of a semi-adjustable articulator would be indicated. Similarly, achieving balanced articulation in a patient with an edentate arch opposed by a natural dentition is facilitated by use of a semi-adjustable articulator. If non-anatomical teeth are used, then a simple hinge articulator will suffice. These issues are discussed in more detail in

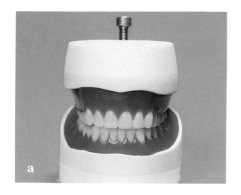

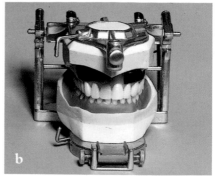

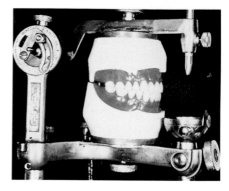

Fig 4-6 Examples of articulators: (a) simple hinge; (b) average value; (c) semi-adjustable.

Chapter 6. In most edentulous cases, using an average value articulator will produce an acceptable result with minimal requirement for chairside occlusal adjustment.

Tips for Registration of the Jaw Relationship – Summary

- Permanent bases can simplify the task of jaw relationship registration.
- Adjustment of occlusal rims should follow a sequential pattern. Appearance requirements dictate the shaping of the maxillary rim. The mandibular rim should then be altered to meet the maxillary rim in centric relation at the planned occlusal vertical dimension.
- Semi-adjustable articulators should be used when balanced articulation with anatomical teeth is planned, or when a complete denture is opposed by a natural dentition.

Conclusions

- Clear prescription of the base material and occlusal rim dimensions should be provided to the dental technician.
- Centric relation is the most reproducible jaw relationship position for complete denture construction.
- Follow all aspects of the treatment plan carefully when adjusting occlusal rims and recording the jaw relationship.

Reference

Academy of Prosthodontics. Glossary of prosthodontic terms. 7th ed. J Prosthet Dent 1999:81;39–110.

Chapter 5
Aesthetic Considerations for Edentulous Patients

Aim

The aim of this chapter is to discuss factors which influence the aesthetics of complete replacement dentures.

Outcome

At the end of this chapter, the clinician should understand that loss of natural teeth and subsequent alveolar resorption has a significant impact on appearance. It is possible to restore appearance with complete dentures, and good communication with the patient is essential. The clinician should understand that aesthetic requirements must be discussed carefully with the patient at the planning stage of treatment. In some cases, it is not feasible to meet the patient's aspirations for the appearance of their dentures, and a compromise must be reached prior to commencement of treatment. The clinician should also make use of reference points such as old photographs or previous dentures with a satisfactory appearance.

Introduction

When natural teeth are extracted, bone volume decreases. Bone resorption in the maxilla occurs mostly on the buccal aspect and this leads to a decrease in lip support. Biometric guides have been described to indicate where the teeth would have been positioned prior to extraction. The reference points are the epithelial band on the crest of the alveolar ridge and the incisive papilla (Fig 5-1). The epithelial band is the remnant of the gingival margins of the teeth, and varies in size. Using these landmarks as a guide, incisor teeth are placed 6 mm anterior to the incisive foramen, and the canine, premolar and molar teeth are placed 8 mm, 10 mm and 12 mm respectively from the epithelial band. In theory, if the denture teeth are placed in these positions, then the appearance of natural teeth can be restored with complete dentures. However, there are a number of aspects to consider when deciding whether to follow these guidelines. Many patients will have been edentulous for many years, and their concept of what constitutes a "normal" appearance may dif-

61

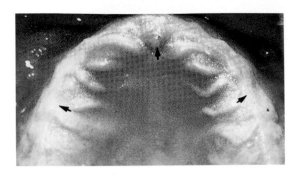

Fig 5-1 Biometric guide landmarks used to indicate position of natural teeth: (a) primary epithelial band and (b) incisive papilla.

fer from that of a dentate patient. When biometric guides are used to guide denture aesthetics, the teeth will appear much more prominent and may not be acceptable to a patient accustomed to a "regular" denture teeth set up. Anthropometric measurements have also been used to guide the selection of anterior teeth for complete dentures. These include dividing the bizygomatic width by a factor of 16, and using the ratio of the cranial circumference to the width of the maxillary anterior teeth (estimated to be 10:1). The concept of relating tooth form to age and sex of the patient has also been used, and this approach suggests that men should have large square teeth, whereas women should have smaller rounded teeth. Certainly, these guides can be useful when the patient has not had dentures before but whether they should be used routinely is questionable.

A further consideration is the impact of tooth position on the retention and stability of the denture. Anterior tooth position also influences speech patterns. Consequently, the approach to designing an aesthetic scheme for complete dentures must be guided by the patient's wishes and functional requirements.

The process of developing an aesthetic scheme for anterior denture teeth begins at the jaw registration stage described in the previous chapter. The wax rims should be adjusted to indicate the desired buccolingual positioning of the teeth and the level of the occlusal plane to the technician. The clinician should check the following when undertaking this task.

Is the patient *satisfied* with the appearance of their previous denture? If the patient has no complaints regarding the appearance of their teeth, then the clinician should aim to copy the appearance in the new dentures. There may be some situations where the clinician may feel that an improvement can be made and this should be discussed at the assessment stage. For example, the clinician can demonstrate the effect of changing the inclination of teeth by using beading wax on the current denture. Aids such as the Alma gauge (Fig 5-2) can also be used to compare occlusal rim inclination with the inclination of teeth on a previous satisfactory denture.

Is the patient *dissatisfied* with the appearance of their previous denture? The clinician should decide what is the source of this dissatisfaction:

- teeth are too large/too small
- too much tooth visible
- not enough tooth visible
- incorrect shade
- unsatisfactory arrangement
- too much gingival display.

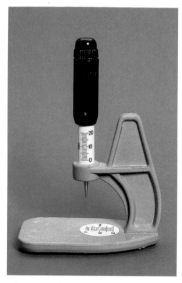

Fig 5-2 Alma gauge. This instrument can be used to measure the distance of the incisal edges of the teeth from the incisive papilla.

In this situation, the clinician must try to find some guide as to how to improve the aesthetics of the new dentures. At the assessment and planning stage, the cause of the dissatisfaction should be elicited. This may be a minor problem, or a source of major dissatisfaction. In the latter situation, it would be helpful if the patient brought some old photographs showing their natural teeth at a subsequent appointment. If they have had a previous denture with an acceptable appearance, this can also be used to guide the aesthetics of the new denture.

Size of the Teeth

There are many mould guides available which help the clinician to choose the size and shape of teeth for a patient. These rely on the clinician's knowledge of the combined width of the six maxillary anterior teeth, and the height and width of the maxillary central incisor. The clinician should choose the mould which most closely resembles these measurements. There is a choice of mould: square, tapering or ovoid (Fig 5-3). In general terms, square moulds suit patients with large, rugged features. Long and narrow faces may be best suited to tapering moulds, whereas ovoid moulds tend to suit patients with

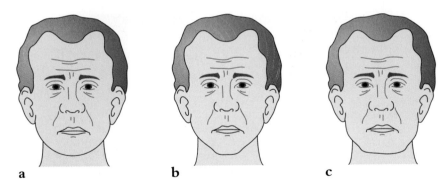

a   b   c

Fig 5-3 Face shapes: (a) ovoid; (b) tapering; (c) square.

small, round faces. The appearance of the old dentures can be helpful in this regard, but if the teeth have worn down then this may not be a particularly good guide. If the old teeth were not aesthetically acceptable, then useful guides include the intercanine lines and the high smile line. The intercanine lines can be marked on the maxillary wax rim by placing an instrument near the inner canthus of the eye, past the ala of the nose and onto the rim (Fig 5-4). This line approximates the position of the distal surface of the canine tooth. The high smile line is obtained by asking the patient to smile broadly and then marking a line on the rim corresponding to the lip position. The distance between the occlusal level of the rim and this line corresponds to the height of the central incisor tooth. The variety of moulds of teeth is limited, and it is occasionally necessary to alter the contour of the teeth with a hand piece.

Shade of the Teeth

Tooth shade is often a source of conflict between the patient and the clinician. There is a tendency for edentulous patients to request bright teeth. Skin colour and tone can be used as a guide, but this may indicate a darker shade than the patient is willing to accept.

Position of the Teeth

The amount of tooth showing, orientation of the occlusal plane, and labi-

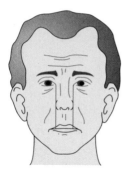

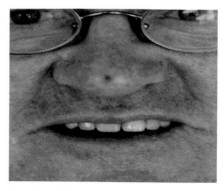

Fig 5-4 Intercanine lines as a guide for anterior mould selection.

Fig 5-5 Unsatisfactory appearance of incisor teeth. They do not follow the smile line and the centre line is too far to the patient's left.

olingual inclination all have an influence on aesthetics. If the level of the occlusal plane is set too low, or if the anterior teeth are set on a flat plane, then the teeth will be too visible. This will be emphasised when the patient smiles, as the teeth will not follow the smile line of the lip. The orientation will also have an influence, and if is not approximately parallel to the interpupillary line, then the smile will look crooked. The centre line of the teeth is also critical, as this will have a negative effect on appearance if it is not coincident with the centre line of the face (Fig 5-5). The labial fraenum should not be used to guide positioning of the centre line, as this is often not in the centre of the face.

The labiolingual position of the anterior teeth, in particular of the necks of the teeth, is critical in terms of lip support. A common misconception is that lip support is reliant on the shape of the labial flange of the denture. However, if the flange is thickened, then this will cause bulking out beneath the nose similar to a gum shield. If teeth are moved away from the crest of the ridge, then this will cause instability of the denture. Setting teeth directly over the crest of the ridge with an upright inclination will not provide adequate lip support. As previously discussed, the use of biometric guides to place the teeth where the natural teeth used to be can improve aesthetics dramatically. A further possibility is to place the necks of the teeth close to the alveolar ridge and tilt the incisal edges of the teeth labially. This will improve the lip support and is less likely to be unstable than when using biometric guides.

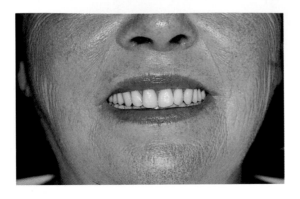

Fig 5-6 Arrangement of teeth to fill the buccal corridor.

Arrangement of the Teeth

In many cases, the patient will request that the teeth are arranged in a regular fashion. However, some patients may wish to reproduce features which were present in their natural dentition. These include spacing, an irregular arrangement and incorporation of restorations in the teeth. Once again, either an old photograph or a previous denture showing these features will be helpful. The photograph, or an impression of the denture should be sent to the dental technician. The shape of the arch of teeth should also be broad enough to reduce the size of the buccal corridor (Fig 5-6) and the inclination of the incisal aspects of the anterior teeth should follow the patient's smile line.

Material of the Teeth

The most routinely used material is acrylic, but porcelain can also be used. Porcelain transmits light in a manner which is similar to natural teeth, and therefore it has good aesthetic properties. It is more resistant to wear than acrylic, and therefore indicated when previous denture teeth have worn quickly. However, there are a number of disadvantages associated with porcelain teeth:
- they do not bond chemically to the denture base
- they are difficult to adjust
- they are noisy.

A number of manufacturers have produced acrylic denture teeth which are available in the full range of Vita porcelain shades. These teeth offer the possibility of excellent aesthetics without the limitations of porcelain teeth.

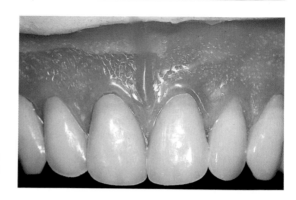

Fig 5-7 Anatomical features reproduced in the appearance of a denture flange.

The Gingival Contour

There are three aspects to consider: (a) the contour of the gingival margins at the necks of the teeth; (b) the contour of the flange; and (c) the colour of the flange. In a natural dentition, the contour of the gingival margin varies from central incisor to lateral incisor to canine. This should be reproduced in a complete replacement denture. In terms of the shape of the flange, the clinician must decide whether to provide a flange with a smooth or anatomical finish. In the case of the latter, the dental technician is instructed to reproduce the shapes of the roots of teeth when contouring the flange. The flange can also be stippled to reproduce stippling of the keratinised gingiva. These features are most useful when the patient has a high smile line and is likely to have a visible flange. A potential problem with anatomical contouring is the difficulty in keeping the flanges clean, particularly when extensively stippled. Finally, the appearance of the oral mucosa can be reproduced using colour tints in the acrylic resin. This is time consuming for a dental technician and will be facilitated by the technician seeing the patient or a photograph of the oral mucosa. Nonetheless, the appearance of the denture will be enhanced if the flange is visible due to a high smile line (Fig 5-7).

Should All Complete Dentures be Class 1?

The incisor relationship in patients with a Class 2 skeletal pattern should have an appropriate degree of horizontal overlap. Failure to provide this will lead to inadequate lip support and problems with articulation of certain speech sounds. It may also be difficult to set the teeth at the correct level, as torquing the teeth into a Class 1 relationship could have the effect of lowering the incisal level. A further important consideration in a patient with a Class 2 skeletal relationship is the positioning of the necks of the mandibu-

67

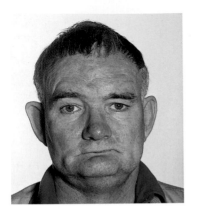

Fig 5-8 Patient with a Class 2 skeletal profile. Note the pronounced mental groove above the prominence of the chin.

lar incisors relative to the lip. Patients with a Class 2 profile tend to have a pronounced mental groove (Fig 5-8), and the action of the mentalis muscle can cause displacement of the denture if the necks of the teeth are too prominent. In patients with a Class 3 skeletal pattern, it may be possible to increase the number of occluding contacts by setting the teeth in a Class 1 relationship. However, in severe Class 3 situations, it is unwise to retrocline the teeth to this extent as the tongue may become cramped. The aim of treatment should be to reduce but not eliminate the reverse horizontal overlap.

Conclusions

- The patient's aspirations for appearance must be determined at the planning stage of treatment, as this will influence contouring of the occlusal rims.
- Whilst many guides are available, there is no substitute for good communication with the patient, and using old photographs or previous dentures with an acceptable appearance for reference.
- In addition to shade and mould, the positioning and arrangement of the anterior teeth are important aspects of denture appearance. The clinician must adjust the occlusal rims to reflect these features and communicate clearly with the dental technician.

Chapter 6
Developing Occlusal Schemes for Complete Dentures

Aim

The aim of this chapter is to discuss the influence of occlusion on the outcome of complete denture therapy.

Outcome

At the end of this chapter, the clinician should be aware that requirements for occlusion in edentulous patients are substantially different from dentate patients. Occlusal schemes for edentulous patients must be developed to facilitate stability and retention of complete dentures. The clinician should be aware that there are a number of occlusal schemes described and the scheme used will influence the choice of posterior teeth. The role of articulators in setting up posterior teeth should also be understood.

Occlusal Schemes – Why Bother?

In Chapter 3, the relationship between retention, stability and support was outlined. A major factor that influences retention is the occlusion of the dentures. The clinician should aim for even, balancing contacts on as many denture teeth as possible during excursive movements. In a dentate patient, the ideal occlusion would be canine guided in excursive movements. If this scheme were incorporated into a complete denture, then the occlusal forces would be directed unilaterally and would overcome forces of retention. The degree of horizontal and vertical (overjet and overbite) overlap of teeth is also relevant. In a patient with a skeletal Class 2 relationship, it may be possible to reduce the amount of horizontal overlap and thus increase the number of occlusal contacts. It is also important to avoid too much anterior overbite, and an edge-to-edge relationship with minimal overbite is the most favourable arrangement (Fig 6-1). However, in some cases, this may affect speech or lead to unsatisfactory appearance. There has been much debate in the scientific literature regarding the impact of occlusion on alveolar resorption. There is little evidence to support the notion that alveolar bone resorption is accelerated by failure to provide balanced articulation. Con-

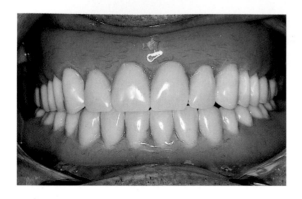

Fig 6-1 Preferred incisal relationship for stability and retention. Note the minimal amount of overlap.

sequently, occlusal schemes for complete dentures should be designed to facilitate:
• denture retention
• chewing.

The emphasis is on the word *designed* as most factors are under the clinician's control.

What Factors Influence Occlusion?

Hanau described five factors which must be considered when developing the posterior occlusion. These are (a) incisal guidance angle; (b) condylar guidance angle; (c) orientation of the occlusal plane; (d) cusp angulation; and (e) slope of the compensating curve. In terms of complete denture construction, with the exception of the condylar guidance angle, all of these factors are under the clinician's control.

The *incisal guidance angle* of the articulator can be set at zero and the teeth placed with minimal overlap. This will decrease or even eliminate incisal guidance during excursive movements, thus reducing tipping forces on the maxillary denture. If cosmetic requirements dictate that a greater degree of overlap between the anterior teeth is required, then the incisal guidance must be greater than zero. As a general principle, when the incisal guidance angle increases, the cusp angle of posterior teeth should also increase to maintain balanced articulation. Once again, this will influence the choice of articulator and a semi-adjustable articulator is indicated when incisal guidance angle is increased.

The *condylar guidance angle* cannot be altered by the clinician as this is related to the path of movement of the condyle in the glenoid fossa during excursive movements of the mandible. It cannot be represented by non-anatomical articulators, and is represented to a limited extent on semi-adjustable articulators.

As described in Chapter 4, the *orientation of the occlusal plane* of complete dentures is dictated by reference to external landmarks such as the interpupillary and the alatragal lines. If the orientation of the occlusal plane is incorrect, then this will impact upon appearance and possibly cause occlusal interferences. The orientation of the plane is determined when shaping the wax occlusal rims during the jaw registration stage and is checked at the trial denture stage.

Cusp angles are determined by the angles of the cuspal slopes to the horizontal plane. As will be described later, posterior teeth come with a variety of cusp angles and the choice of posterior teeth depends on functional and aesthetic requirements.

The *slope of compensating curves* is more relevant for non-anatomical teeth since these can be manipulated to introduce a compensating curve and still maintain balanced articulation. This may improve the appearance of dentures manufactured with cuspless posterior teeth. If substantial compensating curves are introduced into dentures with anatomical teeth, then care must be taken to avoid occlusal disharmony.

Types of Occlusal Scheme

There are many occlusal schemes described for complete dentures, and the choice of the scheme depends mainly on the clinician's preference. Most of these schemes have been developed in an effort to maximise denture stability and retention. Broadly speaking, the schemes can be classified as: (a) balanced articulation; (b) monoplane occlusion; and (c) lingualised occlusion. In the case of *balanced articulation*, the aim is to achieve even contacts between all maxillary and mandibular teeth on the working side (i.e. the side towards which the mandible moves) during excursive movements (Fig 6-2). At the same time, there should be multiple contacts between the mandibular and maxillary teeth on the balancing side (i.e. the side from which the mandible moves) which should not destabilise the denture. The choice of teeth when using this scheme is critical, as it is difficult to avoid tripping cusp contacts with high cusp angle (e.g. 33°) posterior teeth.

71

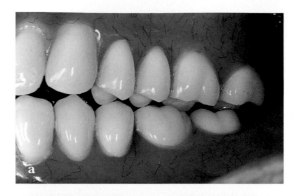

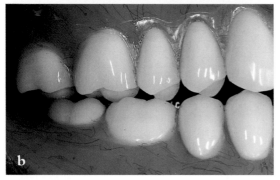

Fig 6-2 Balanced articulation in excursive movements: (a) left side and (b) right side. Note that there is even contact on all posterior teeth.

In the case of *monoplane occlusion*, no attempt is made to create balanced articulation. The occlusal plane is set at the horizontal (Fig 6-3).

Lingualised occlusion involves maximising the contact between the palatal cusps of the maxillary posterior teeth with the central fossae and marginal ridges of the mandibular posterior teeth (Fig 6-4). The buccal aspects of the mandibular posterior teeth are reduced in height and the central fossae are widened to "lingualise" the occlusion. During excursive movements, it is believed that contact between the palatal cusps of the maxillary teeth and central fossa of the mandibular teeth will be maximised thus facilitating stability of the mandibular denture in particular. At the same time, there will be minimal contact between the palatal cusps of the maxillary denture and the buccal aspects of the mandibular denture, thus reducing the potential for tripping.

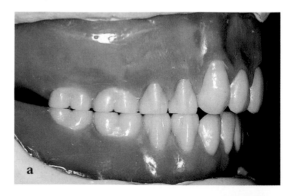

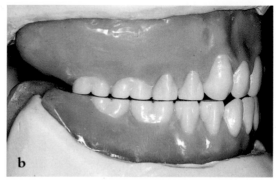

Fig 6-3 Monoplane occlusion: (a) centric relation and (b) protrusion.

Posterior teeth – cuspal inclination

There are four broad categories of posterior teeth:
- Anatomical teeth.
- Non-anatomical (cuspless) teeth.
- Zero-degree cusp teeth.
- Teeth with lingualised features.

Ideally, the teeth used should be *anatomical* as this improves the prospects of the teeth being effective in chewing food. Furthermore, anatomical teeth are also more likely to be aesthetically pleasing than non-anatomical teeth. They are designed to be set up in balanced articulation, and they are available with a variety of cusp angles including 20° and 30°. It is believed that chewing efficiency is likely to be improved with increasing size of cusp angle. Potential problems with anatomical teeth include denture instability when the articulation is not balanced, resulting in trauma to the denture-bearing tissues. This can be particularly problematic if the patient tends to posture

73

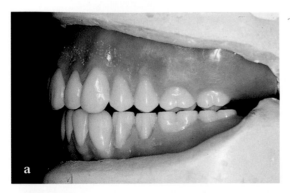

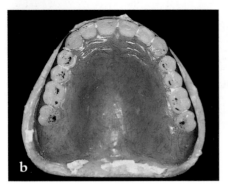

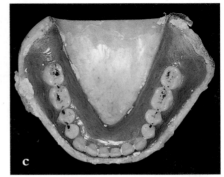

Fig 6-4 (a) Lingualised occlusal scheme with 33° anatomical teeth on the maxillary denture and 10° anatomical teeth on the mandibular denture. Note position of occlusal contacts: (b) maxillary denture and (c) mandibular denture.

the mandible forwards during chewing. The clinician must decide whether the benefits in terms of chewing function outweigh the potential difficulties with anatomical teeth. In addition, the clinician must ensure that anatomical teeth are set up on an articulator which allows excursive movements. If the patient's previous dentures had a wear pattern which was consistent with a ruminative jaw movement, then the anatomical teeth should be set up on a semi-adjustable articulator.

Non-anatomical teeth are designed with flat occlusal surfaces and allow even contact without deflection during excursive movement. They can be used with the monoplane occlusal scheme described earlier, and the teeth can also be set up on a simple hinge articulator. The occlusion is not as badly affected by tooth wear as a balanced occlusal scheme with anatomical teeth is, and thus, in theory, some of the potential disadvantages of anatomical teeth can be avoided. Non-anatomical teeth may also be useful when the alveolar ridge is markedly resorbed and it is difficult to provide a stable mandibular denture. This can be particularly beneficial in patients with reduced capacity for controlling their dentures. However, as non-anatomical teeth do not have cusps, they are relatively ineffective for chewing and patients may experience problems when eating meat or fibrous foods. Some patients may dislike the appearance of these teeth.

Zero-degree teeth have some anatomical features, but have no cuspal slopes. In this regard, they may have some of the advantages of cuspless, non-anatomical teeth without the disadvantages. There is little evidence that they are any more effective for chewing than non-anatomical teeth.

More recently, teeth have been developed for use with lingualised occlusal schemes. They have been designed with the aim of supporting the occlusion with broad contact of the palatal cusps of maxillary posterior teeth with the mandibular posterior teeth. Sluiceways are incorporated to facilitate chewing efficiency. The cusps of the maxillary teeth come in two different sizes, and the shallower cusps are recommended when denture stability and control are problematic.

Posterior teeth – materials

The materials from which posterior teeth are constructed are:
* acrylic resin
* porcelain
* composite resin
* metal onlays (precious or non-precious alloy).

Acrylic resin is the most widely used material for posterior teeth. It offers the advantages of being easy to adjust and bond to the base material. The major disadvantage with acrylic teeth is their relatively poor wear resistance. Porcelain has much better wear resistance, but is difficult to adjust and does not bond to the denture base. Loss of porcelain teeth from the base is a common problem, and patients also complain that the teeth make noise when eating. Composite resin materials are not widely used, but are being used increasingly for complete dentures and implant-retained prostheses opposed by a natural dentition. It is argued that the wear resistance of composite resin is better than that of acrylic composite resin teeth and are easier to adjust and repair than porcelain teeth. Finally, in cases in which the rate of wear acrylic teeth has been extremely rapid, metal onlay restorations can be incorporated onto the acrylic teeth to improve wear resistance. These can be extremely effective, but adhesion of the metal restorations to the underlying acrylic teeth is sometimes a problem.

Conclusions

- Occlusal schemes for posterior teeth in edentulous patients must be developed with the aim of enhancing the stability and retention of complete dentures.
- Posterior teeth can be set up in balanced articulation, monoplane occlusion or lingualised occlusion. There is no evidence that one scheme is more effective than another.
- The choice of occlusal scheme influences the choice of posterior teeth and articulator.
- It is more difficult to achieve occlusal harmony with anatomical teeth than non-anatomical teeth, but anatomical teeth are more aesthetic and are more effective for chewing.
- Acrylic resin posterior teeth are satisfactory, but a more durable material such as porcelain or metal onlays may be indicated when acrylic teeth show signs of rapid wear.

Chapter 7

From Trial Dentures to Delivery

Aim

The aim of this chapter is to describe the assessment of trial and processed dentures.

Outcome

At the end of this chapter, the clinician should be able to decide when trial dentures are ready for processing and delivery to the patient. The clinician should be aware of the requirement for balanced articulation, and that occlusal contacts may need to be altered either at the chairside or with a further laboratory procedure. The patient should also be satisfied with the appearance at this stage. It is imperative that if there are any discrepancies, clear instructions to the dental technician are required to rectify problems. It should also be recognised that after delivery of complete dentures, patients should be provided with clear instructions for the immediate post-delivery stage and given clear instructions on how to clean their dentures. Long-term review is also required.

Assessment of the Trial Dentures

This stage in the denture construction process allows the dentist and patient the opportunity to assess the appearance and occlusion of the dentures prior to processing the bases. If either the appearance or the occlusion of the dentures is unsatisfactory, the problems can be rectified relatively easily at this stage.

The trial dentures should be returned to the surgery on an articulator. The articulated trial dentures should be assessed, and if errors are noted then it is likely that the prescription features of the occlusal rims have not been followed by the technician. The sequence of checks should be the same as the jaw registration stage, starting with the maxillary denture. If the length, position and orientation of the maxillary teeth are correct, these are not changed. The mandibular teeth are then inserted and the occlusion, vertical dimension and freeway space are checked.

Assessment of the trial dentures involves checking the following:
- Appearance of the teeth – This includes size, shade and arrangement of the teeth. The level and orientation of the occlusal plane should also be assessed.
- The positioning of the teeth relative to the neutral zone – Is there any instability associated with the labiolingual positioning of the teeth?
- Is the occlusion balanced? Is there any sign of early contact in centric relation and consequent anterior or lateral slide into the position of maximum intercuspation?
- Is the freeway space correct?
- Phonetics.

Appearance
The patient should be asked for their opinion regarding the appearance of the trial dentures. Assure them that at this stage any aspect can be changed. It may also be helpful to leave them on their own for a few minutes or to invite a friend or relative to give their opinion. Minor alterations can be made at chairside, including changes to the arrangement of the anterior teeth or waxing in the necks of teeth to make them look smaller. Occasionally, the patient will request a different mould or shade of tooth and this will require an extra laboratory and clinical stage. The position of the centre lines should be checked, and if incorrect, then the correct position should be identified and the teeth reset. Orientation of the occlusal plane should be assessed. If it is not parallel with the alatragal and interpupillary lines, the maxillary teeth should be removed and a new jaw relationship recorded.

Tooth position
The maxillary and mandibular trial dentures should be assessed to see if the positioning of the teeth on the rims adversely affects stability. If the maxillary teeth have been set directly over the crest of the alveolar ridge, then the lower teeth are likely to have been set inside the mandibular ridge. This may cause cramping of the tongue (Fig 7-1) and the mandibular denture will rise easily with gentle tongue movements. A further concern would be that the polished surface of the maxillary denture cannot be harnessed to develop a peripheral seal.

In the case of anterior teeth, if these have been set too far forward of the alveolar ridge, instability may be evident. This is seen in patients with a pronounced mental groove or in patients with a very strong mentalis muscle action. If the tooth position is unsatisfactory, the clinician can make minor chairside adjustments by altering the position of the necks of the teeth. If the

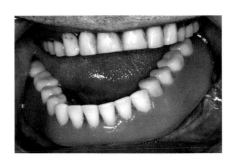

Fig 7-1 Cramping of the tongue. The position of the posterior teeth restricts tongue movement and may destabilise the denture.

occlusion is correct, wax can be added to the buccal aspect of the teeth to indicate to the technician how far buccally the teeth should be moved to correct the error. If the occlusion is incorrect, remove the teeth and reshape the occlusal rims to indicate how both errors should be corrected.

Occlusion

Prior to assessing the occlusion, the clinician should determine that the maxillary denture is satisfactory. Assuming that the maxillary denture is correct, then the mandibular denture can be inserted and the occlusion checked. The occlusion of complete replacement dentures should be balanced, and maximum intercuspation of the teeth should be evident in centric relation. The patient should be guided into centric relation and instructed to bite gently until the teeth first contact. The clinician should stabilise the mandibular trial denture by placing the index fingers on the buccal aspects of the trial denture. If the teeth meet evenly (assuming the freeway space is correct), and the denture teeth slide freely without locking in lateral excursive movements, then the occlusion of the trial dentures is deemed satisfactory. Errors (e.g. Fig 7-2) which may be evident at this stage are:

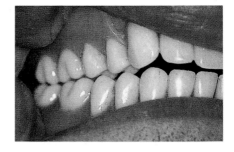

Fig 7-2 An occlusal error evident in trial dentures: posterior teeth meeting too early in centric relation.

- *There is early contact with a slide in an anterior or lateral direction.* This should be suspected if teeth are displaced from the maxillary trial denture. The most likely cause of this is a jaw relationship registration error. This can be confirmed by checking the trial dentures on the articulator – if the teeth meet evenly on the articulator then a jaw registration error should be suspected. Very minor errors may be corrected at the denture delivery stage, as will be discussed later. If a gross error is noted, then the posterior teeth on the mandibular denture should be removed and the jaw relationship re-registered.

- *There is either a unilateral or a bilateral posterior open bite.* In this case, either the level of the teeth in contact is too high, or the teeth out of contact are set too low. If there is too little freeway space, then the problem lies with the level of the teeth in contact. These teeth should be removed, wax should be added to the rim and a new jaw relationship recorded. If the freeway space is correct, then wax should be added to the teeth in the area of the open bite and a new jaw relationship recorded.

- *There is an anterior open bite.* Assuming that the aesthetics of the maxillary denture are acceptable, then check the freeway space. If there is too little freeway space, then the posterior teeth are the cause of the problem, and the lower posterior teeth should be removed and a new jaw registration recorded. If the freeway space is correct and the level of the mandibular anterior teeth is too low, then wax should be added to the anterior teeth to indicate the correct level. The trial denture can then be returned to the dental technician to alter the level of the anterior teeth. A further possibility is to adjust the level of the anterior teeth at the chairside.

If temporary bases have been used, the adaptation of these bases to the underlying tissues should be checked when assessing the occlusion. It is possible that an occlusal interference will displace the bases away from the tissues and give the impression that the teeth meet evenly. This is best checked by placing a flat plastic instrument between the teeth when they are in occluding contact. If the bases are poorly adapted, then a space will appear between the teeth when depressed by the instrument. If this was overlooked at the trial denture stage, then an open bite will be evident on the processed dentures.

Freeway space
The amount of freeway space should be checked by measuring the occluding face height and the resting face height. In addition to measuring the freeway space, the clinician should also assess this visually. If there is too much

tooth showing, or if the patient is struggling to put their lips together, there may be insufficient freeway space. The patient should be asked to speak and if their speech sounds incorrect, this may also indicate that there is insufficient freeway space. It should be borne in mind that problems with speech may also be associated with the retention of the trial denture or thickness of the base if it is too bulky. If there is too much freeway space, then the patient will look overclosed and will show too little tooth.

Phonetics

A number of sounds are affected by tooth position, flange thickness and lip support. The patient should be guided through these sounds during the trial denture stage to assess the effect of tooth position and lip support on phonetics. Some of the problems which may be experienced with speech are listed in Table 7-1. It is sometimes difficult to decide whether phonetics will improve as the patient adapts to the new shape of the dentures. Clinical experience suggests that most patients will adapt. However, the clinician should exercise clinical judgement and make necessary adjustments at this stage if it is considered that the patient is unlikely to adapt to the changes.

Once the trial dentures have been deemed to be satisfactory, they should then be returned to the laboratory for processing. Final instructions to be provided to the technician include the following:
- Position of the postdam.
- Is the acrylic to have a smooth or stippled finish?
- Shading of the gingival acrylic.
- Are deep undercut areas to be blocked out prior to processing the denture base?
- If a permanent soft liner is required, then the technician should be instructed to incorporate this in the denture base.
- Indication of where foil relief is required over areas of poor support such as bony exostoses prior to processing the base.

Table 7-1 Trial denture stage: problems with speech.

Sound	Possible cause
b, p, m	inadequate lip support due to anterior tooth position; lack of freeway space
th	anterior teeth too far forward
f, v	incisal plane of anterior maxillary teeth set too low
s	posterior arch form too narrow; baseplate too thick

81

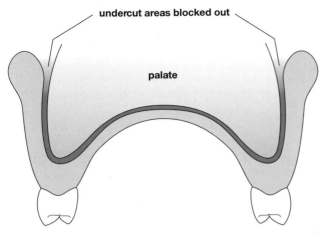

Fig 7-3 Management of undercut areas.

- The material from which the base is to be made, namely standard polymethylmethacrylate (PMMA), high-impact acrylic or metal.
- Incorporation of a reservoir in the denture base for patients with xerostomia.

The position of the postdam should be indicated on the working cast. As a general principle, a smooth finish to the acrylic flange is adequate and may facilitate denture hygiene. However, when the patient has a high smile line, it is appropriate to consider contouring, stippling and staining of the anterior acrylic to mimic the appearance of the attached gingivae and the root form of a dentate patient. This requires a high level of technical skill, but can be very rewarding when executed to a high standard.

When there are pronounced areas of undercut, the technician should be asked to block these out prior to processing the denture base (Fig 7-3). If there is a problem with support for the denture, foil relief over bony exostoses should be provided (Fig 7-4). Resilient lining materials (Fig 7-5) may also be incorporated into the denture base, and, if required, must be prescribed at this time. A resilient lining should be at least 2 mm thick and can be made from plasticised PMMA or heat-cured silicone. Clinical evidence suggests that heat-cured silicone materials are more durable clinically but adhesion to the PMMA base may be a problem. Meticulous hygiene with hypochlorite cleaners prolongs their lifespan, but in view of the clinical limitations of these materials, they should not be considered as first-line treatment.

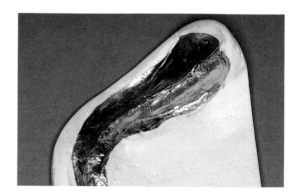

Fig 7-4 Foil relief placed on master cast prior to processing the denture base.

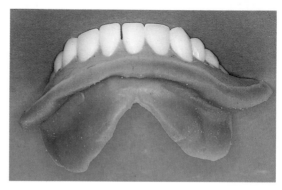

Fig 7-5 Permanent soft lining material incorporated into the denture base.

In some cases, repeated fracture of the PMMA base of a denture cannot be related to poor clinical or laboratory technique and the denture base must be made from a stronger material. Metal bases provide adequate strength, but increase the weight of dentures. High-impact acrylics have proved to function well clinically and have the advantage of being lighter than metal. Incorporation of meshwork into standard PMMA should be avoided, as this concentrates stresses in the acrylic around the meshwork, increasing the risk of fracture.

In patients with xerostomia, a reservoir can be incorporated in the mandibular denture base (Fig 7-6). Lubricating material such as a saliva substitute can be placed in the reservoir and be released gradually into the oral cavity. There is some evidence which suggests that reservoirs increase oral comfort for patients with xerostomia. A potential drawback with reservoir dentures is that they increase the bulk of the mandibular denture and food may also lodge in the opening from the reservoir.

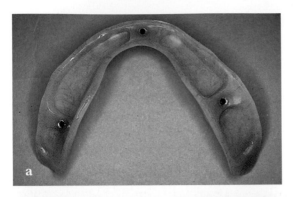

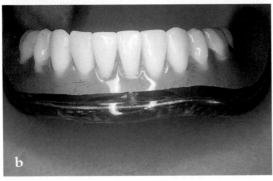

Fig 7-6 (a) Reservoir incorporated into the denture base; (b) fitting surface reattached to the base after a lubricating agent has been placed in the reservoir. (Courtesy of Mr F Nohl)

Delivery of Complete Dentures

Checks on return from laboratory

The dentures should be returned from the laboratory on articulated duplicate casts. When the dentures have been returned from the laboratory, the acrylic should be checked for discrepancies, including:

- Rough or sharp points.
- Scratch marks which indicate poor quality polishing.
- Is the acrylic too bulky or too thin? It should ideally be 3 mm thick.
- Has the plaster been completely removed from the denture?
- Is the contouring of the acrylic satisfactory?
- Has the periphery of the denture been overpolished resulting in loss of the peripheral roll?

If the dentist has a good working relationship with the dental technician, such problems should be infrequent. These problems reflect careless finishing, and should not be tolerated or accepted. If any of these discrepancies are present, they should be corrected before trying the dentures in the patient's mouth.

Final checks

The retention, stability and occlusion of the dentures should be checked prior to delivery of the dentures. Once again the sequence of checks should be the same as for the jaw registration and trial denture stages: check the appearance of the maxillary denture first, determine if it is satisfactory and then check the mandibular denture and the occlusion.

The processed dentures should be retentive, but if they are not, possible causes of poor retention include:

- *Areas of the periphery of the denture are overextended.* This should be suspected if the dentures are initially retentive, but are not retentive if the patient moves their lips/cheeks/tongue. Examine the periphery with the denture in place and look for areas of overextension. It may be helpful to apply pressure-indicating paste (Fig 7-7) to help locate the area of overextension. Once the area of overextension has been relieved, then the denture should become retentive.
- *Areas of the periphery of the denture are underextended.* This should be suspected if the dentures shows no sign of developing a peripheral seal. The most common areas are around the maxillary tuberosities, the distolingual pouch in the mandible and the retromolar pad region. This can be checked by adding green stick tracing compound to the underextended area and muscle trimming. If the denture becomes more retentive, then it should be returned to the laboratory to be rebased to include this further extension.
- *Poor posterior seal in the maxillary denture.* This can be caused by a postdam which is too thick, a postdam which is not on compressible tissue or lack of a postdam. If the postdam is thick, trim this back. This will improve adaptation of the base and should increase retention. If this does not improve retention, then add green stick tracing compound to the posterior aspect of the denture and determine if a posterior seal has developed. If this is successful, then the denture should be returned to the laboratory to add a new postdam. This procedure can also be undertaken using self-cured acrylic resin instead of green stick tracing compound. This has the advantage of avoiding a further laboratory stage, but the self-cured acrylic will show signs of early deterioration.
- *Poor adaptation.* It is clear that when the dentures are not well adapted to the tissues, they are not retentive. This could be due to poor quality definitive impressions or technical errors during the processing of the bases. If

85

a processed base was used during the jaw registration and trial denture stages, then this may have warped when processing the teeth onto the base. When bases are poorly adapted, then the denture will have to be rebased using a procedure described later in the chapter. A further cause of poor adaptation may be the presence of minor bony exostoses on the denture-bearing area (Fig 7-8). If these are identified, the denture should be relieved in these areas until adaptation improves.

- *Poor stability*. This is associated with poor retention and/or occlusal errors. For instance, poor denture stability can be due to the denture displacing mobile tissue or incorrect extension of the bases into the functional sulcus or not extending the mandibular denture over a retromolar pad. It may also be due to occlusal discrepancies, as described next.
- *Occlusal discrepancies*. The dentures should be first checked on articulated casts to assess if there are any discrepancies. The anterior pin on the articulator should remain in contact with the incisal table during excursive movements. Balanced articulation should be evident. When checking the occlusion of the dentures in the mouth, there should be maximum intercuspation in centric relation and no interferences should be present. If articulation is not balanced, a clinical remount procedure should be undertaken. This procedure enables the clinician to assess the lingual aspect of the occlusal contacts as well as the occlusion on the buccal side. The procedure involves the following steps:
  - Record centric relation at a slightly increased vertical dimension. The aim is to have contact only on the registration material and there should be no contact between the teeth with this record. If there is tooth contact, then a new recording should be made. Materials suitable for this purpose include wax or silicone.
  - Record a facebow transfer to allow the upper denture to be mounted on a semi-adjustable articulator.
  - Mount the dentures using the facebow transfer and the interocclusal record on a semi-adjustable articulator (e.g. Denar Mark 3™, Whipmix™); (Fig 7-9).
  - As the pin on the articulator is closed, the interfering contacts will be identified and can be adjusted. Polish the adjusted areas and check the occlusion in the mouth.

Articulating paper may also be used to identify occlusal interferences, but this tends to result in marks on all of the teeth and is therefore not as accurate as a clinical remount. If there are very large errors, then the posterior teeth on the lower denture should be removed and wax added to the base. A new jaw relationship should then be recorded and tried in wax before processing onto the lower base.

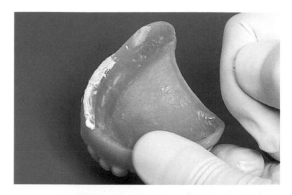

Fig 7-7 Use of pressure-indicating paste to identify areas of overextended denture periphery.

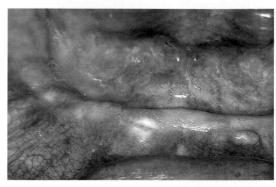

Fig 7-8 Area of inflamed mucosa over bony exostosis. This resulted in poor adaptation of the denture base.

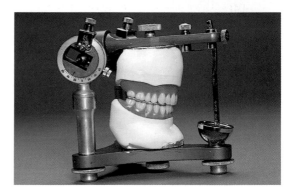

Fig 7-9 Clinical remount of dentures on a semi-adjustable articulator (Dentatus) to refine occlusal contacts.

Post-insertion instructions

The patient may indicate that the new dentures feel strange. They should be advised that this is not unusual. Care should be taken not to alter the new dentures too much at this stage, and time should be allowed for the patient to accommodate to the new dentures. Assure the patient that minor problems are easier to detect following a short period of wearing the dentures and arrange a review visit within one to two days to ensure that there are no major comfort problems. After this, the patient should be reviewed within one or two weeks. The instructions given should include cleaning instructions and what to do in the event of discomfort.

Cleaning instructions
The clinician should take the opportunity to reinforce cleaning instructions. In some cases, it is possible that the patient will receive professional advice regarding denture cleaning and this, of course, is particularly important. The patient should be advised to:

1. Clean the dentures after meals by removing and rinsing them in tap water. A soft bristle brush and warm soapy water can also be used.
2. The dentures should be removed at night time and soaked in a denture-cleaning agent. Denture cleaners can be categorised according to the principal cleaning agent (Table 7-2). There is some debate about their effectiveness, and also concern regarding their effect on permanent and temporary soft lining materials. Hypochlorite solutions appear to cause least damage to soft lining materials, but may bleach acrylic resin and cause corrosion of metal bases. Alkaline peroxide cleaners are probably the most damaging to soft lining materials. The patient should not use toothpaste or hard bristle tooth brushes, as these will scratch the acrylic resin. Furthermore, the dentures should not be soaked in boiling water, as this tends to bleach the denture.

What to do in the event of discomfort
The patient should wear the dentures through the day and should be advised that some minor discomfort is not unusual in the first few days of wear. They should persist with wearing the dentures unless there is extreme discomfort. When the discomfort reaches the extent that the patient cannot eat prop-

Table 7-2 Commonly used denture-cleaning agents.

Agent	Mechanism of action	Examples of brand names
alkaline peroxide	effervescence dislodges foreign material	Steradent™
acid cleaners	softens debris	Denclen™
hypochlorite cleaners	bleaching	Dentural™

erly, then they should remove the dentures and revert to wearing their old dentures. In this situation, it is particularly important that the patient wears the new dentures for a day or so before the recall visit. This will facilitate the identification of the problem areas and allow the clinician to make appropriate corrections to the dentures. Once these instructions have been provided, the patient should be discharged and a review appointment arranged for one to two weeks later. They should take their old dentures home and be advised to store these in a container with a small amount of water to prevent drying and warpage of the acrylic.

How often should the patient be reviewed
There is no consensus on this issue, but it would be appropriate to review the patient at least once per year. If the review period is longer than this, then trauma from the dentures as they become ill-fitting may damage the hard and soft tissues. It also gives the clinician an opportunity to reinforce denture hygiene advice.

Key Clinical Points

- Assess trial dentures in a sequential fashion, starting with the appearance of the maxillary denture. Ensure that the maxillary denture is satisfactory before assessing the mandibular denture and the occlusion.
- Minor problems can be corrected at chairside. Otherwise, the teeth should be reset for a second trial denture stage.
- Follow the same sequence when assessing the processed dentures.
- Review within one to two days of delivery of the denture.
- Annual recall is recommended.

Conclusions

- Trial dentures offer the possibility of detecting and eliminating occlusal discrepancies and patient concerns regarding appearance. Good communication with the dental technician is essential.
- Clear post-insertion instructions regarding the management of discomfort should be given to the patient.
- Denture-cleaning instructions should be reinforced regularly.

Chapter 8
Review Visit: Problem Solving

Aim

This chapter discusses the more common problems associated with new complete replacement dentures and covers their diagnosis and management.

Outcome

By the end of this chapter, the practitioner should recognise that a range of problems may arise with new complete replacement dentures. The cause of these problems may relate to failure of the patient to adapt or to faults in the construction. If a well designed treatment plan has been followed by both the dentist and the dental technician, then many of these problems can be overcome with minor adjustments. Occasionally, a more significant error will become apparent at the first review visit, and this will require more radical alterations and maybe a remake. The practitioner should realise that problems such as pain and looseness may have a single underlying cause, and that eliciting the nature of the problem requires careful discussion with the patient and a thorough clinical examination.

The Review Visit

By the time of the first review visit, the patient should have worn the new dentures for approximately one week. The more common complaints reported include:
- pain/discomfort
- looseness of one or both dentures
- speech problems
- unsatisfactory appearance
- chewing problems.

These problems are not necessarily mutually exclusive, for example pain can be associated with looseness of a denture. It is vital to listen carefully to the patient's account as this is critical to accurate diagnosis and management of the problem. When the patient has outlined their concern, the clinician should conduct a clinical examination and attempt to relate the patient's symptoms to the clinical signs.

Pain/discomfort

This is a particularly common finding with new dentures, and can have many causes.

Overextended periphery. Probably the most frequent aetiological factor is an area of overextension of the periphery. This should be suspected initially if there is an area of well-circumscribed soreness in the sulcus. This may appear as an area of erythema or ulceration of the mucosa. The clinician should relate the area of soreness to the periphery and subsequently adjust the offending area of overextension (as described in Chapter 7). This procedure is facilitated by using pressure-indicating paste (PIP). A small amount of PIP is applied to the suspected area of overextension and dabbed with a sponge. The denture is then reinserted, muscle trimmed and then removed. On inspection, the PIP will have rubbed off in the overextended area. This should be adjusted with a fluted acrylic trimming bur in a straight hand piece and the procedure repeated. When no more PIP rubs off, then the periphery should be polished. Usually, the patient will report instant improvement in discomfort. They should be advised that the soreness may take a day or so to disappear.

Freeway space problem. If there is pain across the entire lower denture-bearing area, then the patient may have too little freeway space. If the patient complains that this pain increases through the duration of the day, then it is almost certainly due to lack of freeway space. Speech may be affected, and further symptoms include unsatisfactory appearance and pain or tiredness in the jaw muscles. Freeway space can be increased by (a) raising the maxillary occlusal plane; (b) lowering the mandibular occlusal plane; or (c) a combination of both. The appearance of the dentures will help determine which of these options to choose. If, for example, there appears to be too much maxillary tooth showing, then option (a) should be chosen and the maxillary denture should be remade. In the case of the patient in Fig 8-1, both mandibular and maxillary dentures were at fault. The denture teeth should be removed from the denture base, a wax rim added and trimmed until sufficient freeway space is achieved. The jaw relationship in centric relation should be registered, and then a trial set-up prescribed in the usual manner. In some cases, there is too much freeway space and this may cause muscular discomfort. This problem will be described in more detail later.

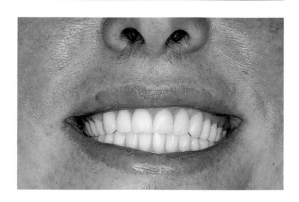

Fig 8-1 Patient with insufficient freeway space. Note, particularly, the level of the mandibular occlusal plane.

Pain in the sulcus. Sometimes, pain and ulceration in the sulcus cannot be attributed to the periphery of the denture. In this situation, the overextension may be in the lingual sulcus and is due to an error in the occlusion. The movement of the denture base, when the lower jaw moves from centric relation to the intercuspal position (ICP) should be noted. If maximal intercuspation is not evident in centric relation, then either a protrusive or lateral slide will occur. If a *protrusive* slide is present, this is likely to cause the denture base to move anteriorly and thus cause trauma to the anterior lingual sulcus. If a *lateral* slide is evident, then contact occurs on one side and the denture base will move to the contralateral side, i.e. a right-sided early contact will result in pain in the left lingual sulcus. If there is a large error (approximately half a tooth out), then the lower posterior teeth should be removed and the jaw relationship re-recorded. If the error is smaller, then clinical remount and adjustment on a semi-adjustable articulator should be undertaken, as described in Chapter 7.

Pain on crest of the alveolar ridge. This may be due to poor quality support tissues or the unemployed ridge phenomenon (described in Chapter 3). Prominent areas of bone have thin mucosa overlying them, and these offer poor support for the denture. They may respond well to relieving the corresponding areas of the denture. Marking the area with an indelible ink or drying the mucosa and applying PIP will help identify the corresponding area on the denture. When the area is sufficiently relieved, the clinician should be able to apply gentle digital pressure to the denture without causing pain. A further possible treatment option is to provide a permanent resilient lining in the denture (described in Chapter 7). Due to the clinical limitations of these materials, this option should be considered as a last resort.

Looseness of one or both dentures

When the patient complains of looseness check (a) peripheral extensions, (b) posterior palatal seal, (c) adaptation of the bases, (d) occlusion, (e) shape of the polished surface and (f) tooth position.

Loose dentures. In the absence of pain and associated overextension of the periphery, looseness of dentures is in all probability a result of a failure to obtain a peripheral seal. A further aetiological factor may be poor adaptation of the denture to the underlying tissues. This should be suspected if the patient complains that food accumulates beneath the denture. The extension of the denture should be checked, and areas of underextension modified with green stick tracing compound. The postdam region of the maxillary denture should also be assessed, and green stick tracing compound added if the postdam is found to be deficient. Common areas for underextension in the mandibular denture are the distolingual pouch and the retromolar pad region.

Another possible cause of denture looseness is that the teeth have encroached upon the neutral zone. If the dentures are unstable when eating and speaking, this is a likely cause. If this is suspected, then the clinician should trim the lingual aspect of the posterior teeth to increase tongue space and assess this after a few weeks. In some cases, there is no major conflict with the neutral zone and the problem is that the shape of the polished surface has been radically altered from that of the previous dentures. These teeth will have to be removed and reset in a position that more closely resembles the previous dentures, and in some cases the dentures will have to be remade.

Denture drops occasionally. In this situation, the denture is reasonably retentive, but occasionally drops without apparent reason. This may be due to a low frenal attachment occasionally displacing the denture. Providing more relief for the frenum may help. A further option is to use a "functional impression" technique. This involves the addition of a resilient material (e.g. Viscogel, Dentsply Ltd, Surrey, UK) to the impression surface of the denture. The patient should then be instructed to undertake functional movements and wear the denture for a few hours. This will allow the full range of the movement of frenal attachments to be recorded. Upon return, the denture should be relined in the conventional way, using the information provided by the functional impression.

The other feature to check is the width of the polished surface around the maxillary tuberosities. When the mouth is opened wide, the coronoid process of the mandible can encroach upon the neutral zone in this region.

If the adjacent polished surface of the denture is bulky, then the denture can be displaced. If this is suspected, then the thickness of the polished surface should be reduced gradually until the patient can open their mouth without displacing of the denture, and the denture polished.

If the impression and polished surfaces are satisfactory, then the problem may be related to the occlusion. Check the occlusion in centric relation and excursive movements. If there is locking of cusps when undertaking excursive movements, then the dentures can be displaced. These contacts should be identified and adjusted until balanced articulation is achieved.

Speech problems

This is sometimes a minor problem. If the patient is not overly concerned, they should be encouraged to resolve the problem by adapting to the shape of the new denture. If the patient has significant difficulty with speech, the areas to check are:

1. The freeway space – If this has been reduced too much, then speech is often affected. The patient frequently complains that they have "a mouthful of teeth". This will have to be addressed as previously described.
2. The thickness of the palatal acrylic – If this is bulky, then the problem may be resolved with reduction of the bulk.

See Table 7-1 in Chapter 7 for potential causes of speech problems related to complete dentures.

Unsatisfactory appearance

It is vitally important to ensure that the patient is happy with the appearance of the dentures at the trial denture stage. However, the patient may have a change of heart following a period of wearing the dentures. This may be due to peer group pressure or unfavourable comments from the family. Often it is due to significant differences between the new and old dentures. The problem may be related to a change in mould or shade of teeth, or to the amount of tooth visible. It may also be related to the inclination of the anterior teeth. Occasionally, the complaint relates to the amount of gingival display. If the retention of the dentures is satisfactory, then alterations can be made without remaking the dentures. The appearance of the old dentures should be used to guide the changes, and it is helpful to record an impression of these for the technician. Changes to the mould, shade or inclination of the teeth can be achieved by removing and replacing the anterior teeth. If the level of the occlusal plane is incorrect, resulting in too much tooth showing or excessive amount of visible polished surface, then all the teeth will have to removed and a new jaw relationship recorded. Wax rims can be added to the denture bases and these should be trimmed to the desired level with reference to the old dentures. When the complaint is that too little tooth is visible, wax can be added to the occlusal surfaces of the teeth until a satisfactory amount of wax is visible (i.e. corresponds to the desired occlusal level). A new centric relation record should be made and the technician should be instructed to remove and reset the teeth to this new position.

Chewing problems

This may present as either an unsatisfactory chewing function or as biting of cheeks or lips when chewing food. If the patient feels that their chewing function has deteriorated with the new dentures, then the following possible causes should be considered:

- The teeth are too flat – If the cuspal angles are too shallow, or if the occlusal surfaces have been adjusted excessively, then the patient may not be able to comminute food properly. Using an interocclusal record, the technician should remount the dentures on an articulator and replace the posterior teeth with appropriate cuspal anatomy.
- Insufficient freeway space – As described earlier, this causes pain in the denture-bearing tissues of the mandible, and chewing problems can be a secondary complaint. There may also be insufficient space to accommodate large amounts of food.
- Excessive freeway space – Add wax to the occlusal surface of one or both dentures to reduce freeway space and record a new jaw relationship. Following a new trial denture stage, process and return the dentures.

If the patient is biting their cheeks or lips when eating, the problem is likely to be due to insufficient horizontal overlap (Fig 8-2). It may be possible to provide some overlap by adjusting the incisal edges or the buccal aspects of the mandibular teeth. A further option is to add a layer of wax to the teeth of the maxillary denture to increase the horizontal overlap and ask the technician to move the maxillary teeth in a buccal or labial direction as indicated by the wax.

To Reline or Rebase?

Assuming that the occlusion is correct, these two procedures can be used to improve adaptation of the denture base to the tissues, and thereby improve retention of the dentures. A reline involves addition of material to the impression surface of the denture, whilst a rebase procedure involves replacing the entire denture base. The reline procedure will increase the bulk and weight of a denture and is more suitable for mandibular dentures than maxillary dentures. A reline can be undertaken either at the chairside or in the laboratory, whereas a rebase procedure involves a laboratory stage. These procedures should be used only when the dentures are reasonably satisfactory: they are not appropriate if there are gross impression or occlusal surface problems. When there is evidence of gross underextension or occlusal wear, then the dentures should be remade. Reline

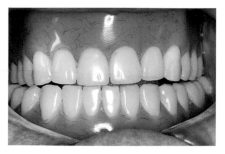

Fig 8-2 Insufficient horizontal overlap of posterior teeth which has caused cheek biting.

or rebase procedures are of value when the tissues have changed shape leading to poor adaptation, but the dentures are otherwise satisfactory. This can occur as a consequence of normal alveolar resorption or volumetric changes in the soft tissues. The latter situation sometimes arises as a consequence of systemic disease and/or medications (e.g. diuretics).

The reline procedure

Check the amount of freeway space present – if it is small, then addition of the reline material may reduce it too much and a remake should be prescribed instead. If there is sufficient freeway space to the extent that loss of 1–2 mm will be of little consequence, then decide whether to undertake a chairside reline or send the denture to a laboratory. Chairside relines have the advantage of speed and are less expensive. However, self-cured reline materials are not as durable clinically and will deteriorate more quickly than heat-cured materials. A number of chairside reline materials are available, however, and the clinical procedure is largely the same for all materials:

- The periphery of the denture should be reduced by approximately 2 mm and any sharp edges removed.
- The adhesive material in the reline kit should be applied, the material mixed according to the manufacturer's directions and then applied evenly to the fitting surface of the denture.
- Place the denture in the mouth and guide the patient into the intercuspal position. Advise the patient that the material may become warm, but will not burn them.
- Keeping the teeth together, muscle trim and allow the material to set.
- When the material has set, remove and inspect the denture. There should not be any defects in the set material – if there are, remove the reline mate-

rial and repeat the procedure. If satisfactory, remove any sharp edges and polish.

If it is decided that the reline should be done in the laboratory, then the following steps are undertaken in the clinic:
- The denture periphery should be adjusted to allow approximately 1 mm thickness of impression material.
- Apply adhesive to the impression surface of the denture, taking care to apply adhesive to the periphery.
- Apply a medium viscosity polyvinylsiloxane material to the impression surface. Insert the denture and guide the patient into the intercuspal position. Muscle trim and allow the material to set.
- Remove the denture, inspect and if satisfactory, send to the laboratory with a prescription for a heat-processed reline.

The rebase procedure

As mentioned earlier, a rebase procedure is more appropriate for the maxillary denture. The clinical stages are the same as those described above for the laboratory reline procedure. The periphery of the denture is relieved by approximately 2 mm, and any undercuts in the denture base removed. Using a closed-mouth impression technique, an impression is recorded in polyvinylsiloxane and sent to the laboratory with instructions to rebase the denture.

Conclusions

- If a well designed treatment plan has been implemented, then the adjustments required at the first review visit should be minimal.
- Occasionally, problems may arise which require more substantive adjustments. These may sometimes require further laboratory procedures.
- The occlusion is pivotal to denture retention and stability and its importance is often underestimated. Always remember to check occlusion when there are retention and comfort problems.
- Reline or rebase procedures are occasionally indicated but should not be used as a panacea for poor denture construction technique.
- Edentulous patients should have long-term review appointments to monitor the health of the oral mucosa.

Chapter 9
Building On Success with Copy Dentures

Aim

The aim of this chapter is to discuss the use of the replica or copy denture technique.

Outcome

The polished surfaces of complete dentures can be harnessed to facilitate physiological retention. The clinician should understand the indications for the use of the copy technique and realise its limitations.

Introduction

The issue of patient adaptation to complete replacement dentures has been discussed in Chapter 1. In general, the ability to adapt to change diminishes with age. A key element identified in helping the patient to adapt is the shape of the polished surface of the denture. If the patient has had a set of complete dentures for many years, then they will probably have used their ability to control the dentures with their orofacial musculature to overcome loss of adaptation to the tissues. If the clinician substantially changes the shape of the polished surface, then the patient may not be able to control the new dentures. For this reason, the clinician should duplicate the shape of the old dentures where possible. One technique employed for achieving this is the "copy technique".

Copy Technique – Rationale

The purpose of the copy technique is to reproduce as closely as possible the polished surface shape of the old dentures in the new dentures. The principal changes in the new denture will be to the impression surface and occlusal surfaces. The technique involves recording an impression of the denture which is then used to produce a replica or template. The replica is then used in the clinical and laboratory stages of replacement denture construction.

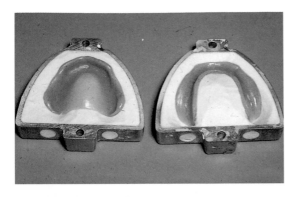

Fig 9-3 Copy denture technique: use of aluminium flasks to make impressions of the dentures. (Courtesy of Mr ID Murray)

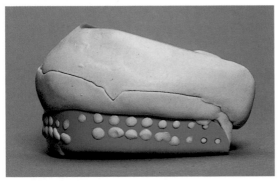

Fig 9-4 Copy denture technique: use of impression putty to make an impression of the denture. (Courtesy of Mr ID Murray)

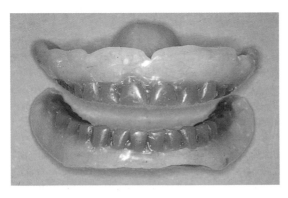

Fig 9-5 Self-cured acrylic replica with wax teeth. (Courtesy of Mr ID Murray)

tion form for the dental laboratory should be completed. This should include the material to be used for construction of the replica, that is, wax for the teeth and self-cured acrylic resin for the base (Fig 9-5) or self-cured acrylic resin for the teeth and the base. When a trial denture is required, the clinician should prescribe the mould and shade for the teeth.

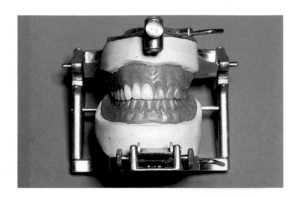

Fig 9-6 Trial set-up for copy denture technique. (Courtesy of Mr ID Murray)

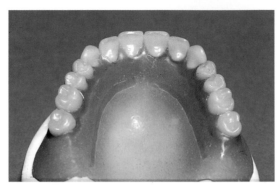

Fig 9-7 Preparation of "slots" on the base prior to return to the clinic. (Courtesy of Mr ID Murray)

Producing the replicas

Once the replicas have been produced, they are mounted on the articulator. The technician removes the wax (or acrylic) teeth one by one from the replicas and gradually a set of trial dentures is produced (Fig 9-6). This procedure is facilitated by using a stone model of the teeth cast from the replica impressions. The technician should incorporate "slots" in the base of the replicas prior to returning the trial dentures to the clinician (Fig 9-7).

Trial denture stage

When the trial dentures are returned to the clinician, the occlusal relationship should be checked. There should be balanced articulation with an acceptable freeway space. The appearance should be checked to see if the patient is satisfied with the colour, shape and arrangement of the teeth. Minor changes can be made at the chairside, whereas major changes may require a retry visit. When the trial dentures are deemed acceptable, then definitive impressions are required.

Definitive impression procedures

The extension of the replicas should be checked: areas of overextension must be trimmed back to allow an adequate thickness of impression material in the sulcus area. If the bases are underextended, then green stick tracing compound should be added to correct the extension of the periphery. The working impressions are recorded using a closed-mouth impression technique. This is required to avoid disrupting the occlusal scheme. The impression material chosen is largely the operator's choice. Zinc oxide and eugenol paste and low viscosity elastomer materials are commonly used for this purpose. If the amount of freeway space is small (3 mm or less), then a paste impression material is preferred to avoid inadvertently losing too much freeway space.

The impressions for each jaw should be recorded separately. The sequence of events, starting with the maxillary denture, are as follows:

1. Remove undercuts from the replicas. This will facilitate removal of the replicas from the working casts once the definitive impressions have been cast.
2. Place impression material in the maxillary replica.
3. Seat the replica in the mouth, ensuring that it is fully seated.
4. Place the mandibular replica in the mouth and ask the patient to close gently. The replicas should meet evenly.
5. The tissues should be manipulated with the replicas held together to develop the shape of the periphery. Support the jaw while the impression material sets (Fig 9-8).
6. Remove the replicas and check that the impression is satisfactory.
7. Reseat the maxillary replica, and add impression material to the mandibular replica.
8. Place the mandibular replica in the mouth, and ask the patient to close gently. The replicas should meet evenly.
9. Repeat the muscle trimming procedure as for the maxillary impression, including asking the patient to swallow. Support the jaw while the impression sets.
10. Remove the replicas and check that the impression is satisfactory.

The technician casts the impressions and prepares the replicas for flasking and packing.

Modified Copy Technique

The copy technique can also be used to construct dentures incorporating significant differences from the pretreatment dentures. In addition to chang-

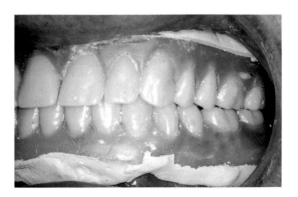

Fig 9-8 Recording of definitive impressions with zinc oxide and eugenol paste using the closed-mouth technique. (Courtesy of Mr ID Murray)

ing the impression surface, major changes can also be made to the occlusal surfaces. In this situation, the replicas should be constructed with wax teeth and a jaw registration stage undertaken. The production of the replicas is as previously described. Wax is added to the replicas until even contact is achieved in the planned occluding vertical dimension with the planned freeway space. If appropriate, the shape of teeth can also be changed by adding wax to the labial aspects of the teeth or removing wax from the lingual or palatal aspects. The replicas should then be sealed together. Once a shade of tooth has been chosen, the replicas should be returned to the laboratory and teeth set up for a trial denture procedure. The trial denture stage should be undertaken as previously described.

Indications

The copy technique is used mainly for older adults who have had a set of complete dentures for many years and for whom adaptation to new dentures may be difficult. This technique can also be used to construct new dentures for patients whose neuromuscular control has been compromised by disease. This includes patients with Parkinson's disease and patients who have had a stroke. By copying the polished surface shape of a previous set of dentures, adaptation to new dentures may be facilitated.

Drawbacks

In theory, it is possible to use the copy technique for any complete denture replacement. However, one should be wary of using this technique to replicate technically inadequate dentures. For instance, when maxillary teeth have been placed directly over the crest of the alveolar ridge, then it is likely that

105

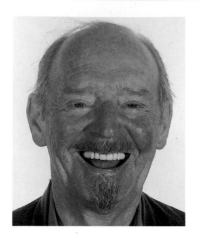

Fig 9-9 Use of the copy technique has produced a maxillary denture with narrow arch form. A replacement technique would have allowed greater flexibility in tooth arrangement.

there is a poor peripheral seal. By copying this polished surface, the shape of the new denture will not be harmonious with the facial tissues (Fig 9-9) and physical retention of the denture will be compromised. Control of the working impression is also reduced when using a closed–mouth impression technique, and this could be critical in situations where the denture-bearing area is unfavourable. For instance, if the maxillary ridge has been replaced by flabby tissue, then the compressive impression technique may displace this tissue leading to an unstable denture.

Conclusions

- Preserving the shape of polished surfaces in new dentures may help a patient to adapt to new dentures.
- The replica technique can be used to copy the shape of the polished surface of old dentures.
- This technique can be of great benefit when constructing dentures for elderly patients, or patients with neuromuscular deficits.

Chapter 10

The Shifting Treatment Paradigm: Replacement Dentures or Implant-retained Prostheses?

Aim

The aim of this chapter is to discuss the influence of osseointegrated dental implants on treatment planning for edentulous patients.

Outcome

At the end of this chapter, the practitioner should be aware of the potential benefits of implant-retained prostheses in the rehabilitation of edentulous patients. However, it should also be recognised that provision of implants may not be straightforward, and that anatomical and financial restrictions may complicate treatment. Furthermore, older adults may not wish to undergo a complex form of treatment, especially one which involves surgery. Although the benefits of implants in retaining oral prostheses are obvious, the burden of maintenance is high and something which should clearly be considered and built into the treatment plan. The clinician should consider the merits of implant overdentures retained on two implants in the mandible for older adults.

Introduction

The outcome of complete replacement dentures is variable and is dependent on the patient's ability to overcome the limitations of dentures. The advent of osseointegrated implants has dramatically improved the options for edentulous patients. The use of implants to stabilise prostheses reduces the need for the patient to develop the complex skills required to control complete dentures. Potentially, this can help improve oral function for the patient. Furthermore, it is possible to achieve greater patient satisfaction with the appearance of complete dentures which are retained on dental implants. The term "implant-supported prostheses" refers to intraoral prostheses which are entirely supported on osseointegrated dental implants. The term "implant-retained prostheses" may also be used, and these terms are often used interchangeably. It may be argued that the latter term is more appropriate for an intraoral prosthesis which shares its support between the oral

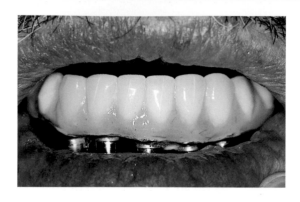

Fig 10-1 Mandibular implant-retained bridge.

mucosa and dental implants. Such a prosthesis is commonly referred to as a "hybrid prosthesis". In all cases, prostheses are "stabilised" by implants.

Fixed Implant Prostheses

Two types of complete (as opposed to partial or single tooth) prosthesis are described: (a) a fixed bridge; and (b) a removable overdenture. The fixed bridge prosthesis (superstructure) is connected to the implants (also known as fixtures) via a transmucosal abutment assembly, as shown in Fig 10-1. The prosthesis is held in place using either screws or a dental cement. In the mandible, the prosthesis is supported by four to six implants in the anterior mandible. These fixtures are placed between the mental foramina to avoid damaging the inferior dental and mental nerves. The length of the implants used is determined by the height of jaw bone available, as determined from preoperative panoramic radiographs. The distal extensions of the prosthesis are cantilevered backwards from the most posterior fixtures. At least eight implants are required to support a fixed bridge in the maxilla, as bone quality and quantity is inferior to that found in the mandible. The site of implant placement is influenced by anatomical structures such as the floor of the nose and maxillary air sinuses.

Removable Implant Overdentures

Where the number of implants which can be placed is restricted, a removable overdenture may be used. This type of prosthesis may be entirely supported by implants, or may share its support between implants and oral mucosa. In the first instance, a precious metal alloy bar is attached to the implants (three to four in the mandible, at least six in the maxilla) via a trans-

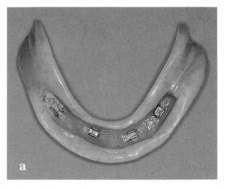
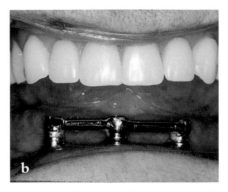

Fig 10-2 Implant overdenture on a long bar. (a) Metal clips in the fitting surface; (b) long bar retained on three fixtures.

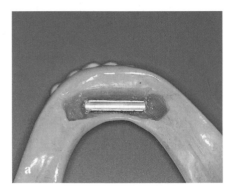
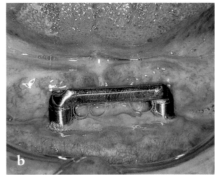

Fig 10-3 Implant overdenture on a short bar. (a) Metal clips in the fitting surface; (b) short bar retained on two fixtures.

mucosal abutment assembly (Fig 10-2). The denture is attached to the bar using metal clips embedded in its impression surface. Where support is shared between implants and mucosa, the prosthesis is retained either using a short precious metal bar (e.g. Dolder bar) and clips (Fig 10-3), or ball attachments and rubber "O" rings (Fig 10-4). This type of prosthesis is indicated where prosthesis retention is the most significant problem, and has the advantage of being less expensive than the long bar overdenture and fixed bridge options. It is less useful when the denture-bearing area provides poor support for a denture. This is likely to be the case if there is very little keratinised gingiva and if mental nerve compression is evident clinically. In this situation, either a fixed bridge or a long bar overdenture is indicated.

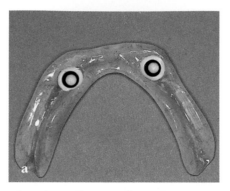 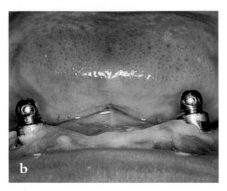

Fig 10-4 Ball-retained overdenture. (a) "O" rings in the fitting surface of the denture; (b) ball attachments on two fixtures.

Planning which prosthesis design to use is influenced both by patient preference and by the quantity and quality of bone available. In the case of the former, a careful discussion with the patient is advised to ascertain exactly what they desire from their treatment. Bone levels should be assessed preoperatively by radiographic means. Guidelines for assessment of bony ridge quality and quantity have been described by Lekholm and Zarb (1985) and Cawood and Howell (1991).

Complete Replacement Dentures or Implants?

There is a growing shift towards the routine use of implants to stabilise complete removable prostheses. This is driven by the fact that implants can overcome many of the functional, psychological and physiological consequences of edentulousness. Implants help to preserve alveolar bone and bite force is increased when compared with conventional complete dentures. This may enable the patient to chew food with a higher nutritional value and this, in turn, is important for general health. However, they are more expensive and complicated to provide that conventional dentures, and a number of factors need to be considered when planning implant-retained dentures.

What are the patient's concerns?

If the edentulous patient has unmet expectations, then implant-retained prostheses can be of great benefit. However, if the patient is seeking a replacement of their own natural dentition "like with like", then these expectations are unlikely to be met. A further consideration is whether a removable or fixed prosthesis is chosen. There is some evidence that both types of prosthesis are equally effective in restoring oral function, but patients may express a preference. The advantage of using a removable overdenture is that fewer implants are required and financial costs are decreased. Unlike a fixed bridge prosthesis, tissue support by way of a flange can also be provided with a removable prosthesis. However, there are maintenance costs associated with implant-retained prostheses and these appear to be higher with removable overdenture prostheses. Commonly reported problems include loosening of components, fracture of gold alloy screws and the need for replacement of retention clips.

Are implants feasible?

The provision of implants must be planned jointly by the surgeon and the prosthodontist. The level of bone should be assessed in terms of the width and height of alveolar ridge present. A number of anatomical landmarks such as the maxillary antra, floor of the nose and inferior dental nerve influence the positioning of implants. Whilst panoramic radiographs are appropriate for assessing the possible implant sites, the use of a computerised tomography (CT) scan is sometimes indicated. This allows a three-dimensional view of the bony ridge and increases the accuracy of treatment planning. The attached mucosa should also be assessed and if there is very little of this left, then an implant-retained prosthesis should be supported entirely by implants.

Generally the patient should be fit enough to undergo minor oral surgery and be willing to be involved in a lengthy course of treatment. Patients who smoke should be advised that the failure rate of implants is much higher in smokers than non-smokers.

There are few absolute medical contraindications to implant-retained prostheses, and these include:
• any condition that precludes a minor oral surgical procedure (e.g. poorly controlled diabetes mellitus, blood dyscrasias, immunologically compromised)
• history of chemical dependency
• recent history of orofacial radiation
• unstable psychiatric disorders
• heavy smoking.

Should implants be placed in one or both jaws?

Clinical experience and research findings indicate that most denture problems are associated with mandibular complete dentures. In many cases, patients are satisfied with maxillary dentures. Consequently, a complete replacement denture in the maxilla opposed by an implant overdenture in the mandible is likely to satisfy the patient's requirements. This simplifies treatment and reduces cost.

Fixed or removable prosthesis

Studies indicate that fixed and removable implant prostheses are equivalent in terms of improvement in oral function. Some patients may prefer to have a fixed prosthesis, but they should be aware of certain limitations. It is almost impossible to restore appearance to a pre-extraction level with a fixed prosthesis, particularly in the maxilla. Phonetics is also affected by the escape of air between the abutments in maxillary prostheses. Furthermore, when a mandibular fixed prosthesis is opposed by a maxillary complete denture, patients often report that their maxillary denture is less retentive in function. Given these limitations, it is important that the treatment plan matches the patient's aspirations and that the fixed prosthesis is not seen as a gold standard for implant prostheses.

When is it Appropriate to Refer?

With suitable training, implant overdentures can be provided in general dental practice. It is vitally important that the practitioner who provides the overdenture directs the surgical stage of treatment. It is not good practice to conduct surgical and restorative phases of treatment independently, and major difficulties arise when the surgeon and prosthodontist do not communicate clearly with each other. When a general dental practitioner is deciding whether to refer the patient to a specialist practitioner for an opinion regarding the possibility of having implants, the following points should be considered:

- Has the patient had any complete dentures?
- Have deficiencies with current dentures been addressed?
- Do they understand what implants involve?

If the existing dentures are grossly deficient, then there is little justification in immediately seeking an implant consultation. It may be possible to overcome the difficulties using conventional replacement dentures and these should be constructed in the first instance. Occasionally, the patient may request extraction of their remaining natural teeth and an immediate replacement retained on implants. If the patient has never had complete or partial dentures, then a number of potential difficulties arise. The clinician does not know for certain what freeway space is required for that patient, or whether

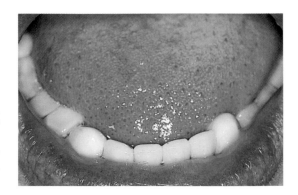

Fig 10-5 A patient provided with bilateral, posterior implant-retained prostheses. As a consequence of tongue cramping, it has not been well tolerated.

there is sufficient neutral zone to accommodate posterior teeth (Fig 10-5). In this situation, the patient should have complete dentures made as a diagnostic procedure. This allows the clinician to determine the correct position of teeth and subsequently where the implants should be placed. Finally, the patient should understand that implant therapy involves:

- At least one and possibly two surgical stages. The traditional approach to providing implants involves a two-stage surgical procedure. In the first-stage surgery, the fixtures are placed and then covered for four to six months to allow time for osseointegration. The second stage involves uncovering the fixtures and preparing the implant site for the prosthetic phase of treatment. More recently, a one-stage approach has been described. This involves early loading of implants in the mandible, and this has the advantage of shortening the treatment process. Short-term research reports have been favourable, and a one-stage approach may become the norm in the future.
- The patient will have to avoid wearing their denture during the first one to two weeks after surgery. They may also have to have their denture modified during the surgical healing phase.
- Failure of implants is possible. This includes failure of the implants to osseointegrate and long-term failure.
- There is a burden of maintenance associated with implant-retained prostheses. This includes maintenance of plaque control (Fig 10-6) and mechanical maintenance. Adjustment and repair of components is not unusual and the patient needs to understand this in advance.
- There are substantial costs associated with implant therapy.

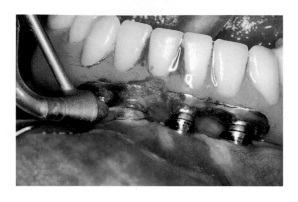

Fig 10-6 Poor oral hygiene procedures have led to gingival inflammation. Ongoing maintenance procedures are required.

Conclusions

- Implant-retained prostheses have been a major advance in the treatment of patients with denture-wearing difficulties, and offer the possibility of overcoming the problems associated with conventional replacement dentures.
- Provision of implant-retained prostheses involves surgical and prosthetic phases and must be planned jointly by the surgeon and prosthodontist.
- Referral of patients to specialists should be contemplated only when deficiencies in the conventional dentures have been rectified.
- There is a lifetime burden of maintenance associated with implant-retained prostheses and the patient should be aware of this prior to commencing treatment.

Further Reading

Branemark PI, Albrektsson T, Zarb G. Tissue Integrated Prostheses: Osseointegration in Clinical Dentistry. Chicago: Quintessence, 1985.
Cawood JI, Howell RA. Reconstructive preprosthetic surgery. I. Anatomical considerations. Int J Oral Maxillofac Surg 1991;20:75–82.

Index

Quintessentials for General Dental Practitioners Series

in 36 volumes

Editor-in-Chief: Professor Nairn H F Wilson

The Quintessentials for General Dental Practitioners Series covers basic principles and key issues in all aspects of modern dental medicine. Each book can be read as a stand-alone volume or in conjunction with other books in the series.

Publication date,
approximately

Oral Surgery and Oral Medicine, Editor: John G Meechan

Practical Dental Local Anaesthesia	available
Practical Oral Medicine	Spring 2004
Practical Conscious Sedation	Autumn 2003
Practical Surgical Dentistry	Spring 2004

Imaging, Editor: Keith Horner

Interpreting Dental Radiographs	available
Panoramic Radiology	Autumn 2003
Twenty-first Century Dental Imaging	Autumn 2004

Periodontology, Editor: Iain L C Chapple

Understanding Periodontal Diseases: Assessment and Diagnostic Procedures in Practice	available
Decision-Making for the Periodontal Team	Autumn 2003
Successful Periodontal Therapy – A Non-Surgical Approach	Autumn 2003
Periodontal Management of Children, Adolescents and Young Adults	Autumn 2003
Periodontal Medicine in Practice	Spring 2004

Implantology, Editor: Lloyd J Searson

Implants for the General Practitioner	available
Managing Orofacial Pain in General Dental Practice	Spring 2004

Endodontics, Editor: John M Whitworth

Rational Root Canal Treatment in Practice	available
Managing Endodontic Failure in Practice	Autumn 2003
Managing Dental Trauma in Practice	Autumn 2003
Managing the Vital Pulp in Practice	Autumn 2004

Prosthodontics, Editor: P Finbarr Allen

Teeth for Life for Older Adults	available
Complete Dentures – from Planning to Problem Solving	Autumn 2003
Removable Partial Dentures – A Systematic Approach	Autumn 2003
Fixed Prosthodontics for the General Dental Practitioner	Autumn 2003
Occlusion: A Theoretical and Team Approach	Autumn 2004

Operative Dentistry, Editor: Paul A Brunton

Decision-Making in Operative Dentistry	available
Applied Dental Materials in Operative Dentistry	Spring 2003
Aesthetic Dentistry	Autumn 2003
Successful Indirect Restorations in General Practice	Spring 2004

Paediatric Dentistry/Orthodontics, Editor: Marie Therese Hosey

Child Taming: How to Cope with Children in Dental Practice	Spring 2003
Paediatric Cariology	Autumn 2003
Treatment Planning for the Developing Dentition	Autumn 2003

General Dentistry and Practice Management, Editor: Raj Rattan

The Business of Dentistry	available
Risk Management in General Dental Practice	Autumn 2003
Practice Management for the Dental Team	Autumn 2003
Application of Information Technology in General Dental Practice	Spring 2004
Quality Assurance in General Dental Practice	Autumn 2004
Evidence-Based Care in General Dental Practice	Spring 2005

Quintessence Publishing Co. Ltd., London